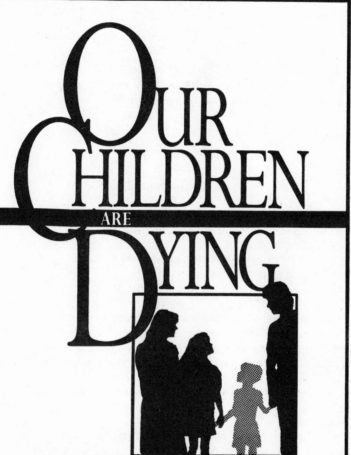

OUR CHILDREN ARE DYING

RECOGNIZING THE DANGERS AND KNOWING WHAT TO DO

MARIETTA P. STANTON, Ph.D., R.N.

with a contribution by Wanda Therolf, Attorney at Law

PROMETHEUS BOOKS
BUFFALO, NEW YORK

This book is dedicated to my six-year-old brother Brian, who died many years ago as the result of a drunk driver's negligence, and to my brother Buddy, who never got over it—I remembered!

Published 1990 by Prometheus Books

Editorial offices located at 700 East Amherst Street, Buffalo, New York 14215, and distribution facilities at 59 John Glenn Drive, Amherst, New York 14228

Library of Congress Cataloging-in-Publication Data

Stanton, Marietta P.
    Our children are dying : recognizing the dangers and knowing what to do / by Marietta P. Stanton.
        p.   cm.
    Includes bibliographical references.
    ISBN 0-87975-609-8
    1. Children—United States—Mortality. 2. Child abuse—United States. I. Title.
HB1323.C52U67   1990
362.7′1′0973—dc20
                                                                                            90-8910
                                                                                            CIP

Printed on acid-free paper in the United States of America

Contents

5

Preface

It is often said that the quality of life in the future lies with our children. If this is true, then the time and energy we give to our smallest citizens will reward society for years to come. Many people will point to the progress that has been made in health care, social programs for children, and reforms in child-welfare regulations and proclaim that our children's lives are secure and happy. It is true that in the past century many programs for children have developed, but do they really protect our kids? Have they had much success? Can they do it all? For that matter, should we expect them to? What role should we as adults play to assure a happy, healthy childhood for all our children?

This book will attempt to answer these questions, at least in part; it will assess where we are and where we need to go to ensure that every child has a chance to grow and succeed in life. It is not intended just for parents but for all adults, because all adults share this responsibility whether they happen to be parents or not. To paraphrase a line from Genesis, "We are our brother's keeper." We share a solemn obligation to protect the best part of our heritage, our children, and to pass that legacy of loving concern and compassion on to future generations.

We needn't look very far to discover the extent to which we are failing our children: local and national television news reports, network specials, radio news and talk shows, as well as local and national newspapers daily report the young victims of tragic situations. From Sudden Infant Death Syndrome (SIDS) and skyrocketing infant mortality to accidental poisonings and drug or alcohol-related deaths, from backyard pool drownings to prom-night head-on collisions, from child abuse to teenage homicide and suicide, the list of problems that threaten to snuff out precious young lives is growing at an alarming rate and the national death-toll is rising. How much potential greatness has already been lost to us? The death of a child represents a unique contribution to society that can never be realized. As each special child dies, we lose another chance to make our lives, our country, and our world a better place. Trite as it sounds, children are our most precious resource; they are diamonds in the rough that we love, nurture, and polish to replace us.

Children are our mirrors. They reflect the love and care we have given them. Can we look in that mirror and feel happy and content with what we see? Sometimes it seems we can. Parents watch their child march up to receive a kindergarten diploma. The youngster's face is all smiles, and this is a very proud moment for parents and child alike. But at other times we see a face that shows the signs of abuse, the lack of medical care, or the ravages of poverty. It then becomes very difficult for adults to look in that mirror. We can pretend that these reflections of ourselves are very infrequent. But are they?

Historically, the United States has been concerned with the welfare and happiness of its children: the existence of many federal, state, and local statutes and publicly funded programs prove this. In addition, volunteer organizations such as the Children's Defense Fund or the March of Dimes have been concerned with children and the quality of their lives. However, on examining the evidence, it's hard to ignore the fact that we lose many children every year. This country is a rich and successful nation, yet not all of our children benefit from this wealth. The United States, in recent years, has not done as much as it should to prevent social and health problems that claim our children as victims. Many children do not have an opportunity to get medical help before problems result in serious illness or death. The poor have limited access to routine medical checkups. The bottom line is that preventing major health problems can benefit a child for a lifetime, while denying care can increase the likelihood of illness, disability, and death.

But this is just one facet of a very complicated issue. Poverty and its devastating consequences account for only a portion of the childhood deaths reported each year. Even children who seem to have every advantage in life—the best of everything—die unnecessarily. If we were to set aside the risks that stem from socioeconomic conditions, our youngsters would still be in jeopardy. Each age level experiences its own special set of risk factors, its own obstacles for both parent and child. No adult can turn away from these childhood deaths with the secure assurance that "this doesn't affect me, my child's not at risk." *All children are at risk.* Since no child is entirely safe, adults must confront the facts and find ways to protect the children in their care.

In the course of my research on the causes of death in infants, young children, and adolescents, I spoke to many parents, friends, and neighbors. I was shocked and alarmed to find that all but a few had experienced some tragedy with their own child or with a young person who had been close to their family or friends. One neighbor's child had died in infancy from SIDS. The teenage son of a close personal friend died in a bicycle accident. Another had a son who committed suicide when he was a high school senior. These are just a few examples. The fact that this carnage seems to be accepted as part of normal life for today's parents is a frightening comment on the status of children in our society. We not only sense the tragedy of it all but we are anguished at our failure as adults to prevent childhood death.

The problem of dying children was also very evident in all that I read. Each study and interview strengthened my commitment to get to the heart of this problem and to find ways to prevent these senseless tragedies. One of the goals of this book, therefore, is to offer a comprehensive overview of the ways children die at various ages and to suggest the reasons for these deaths. My aim is not to make adults feel guilty or uncomfortable (though many should) but to isolate the causes of these tragedies so that individual parents and citizens can initiate actions to prevent future deaths.

Understanding the causes of death among our nation's youth is a valuable step in the right direction, but it is also vitally important to know what is being done to safeguard our young people and to determine if these methods are achieving their goals. What are the characteristics of an effective method, and what features spell failure? Perhaps in finding these answers we may be in a better position to develop solutions appropriate to our present and future needs.

It is clear that parents, grandparents, and close family should be on the front line of prevention. However, as anyone who has worked with children knows, this is often an ideal to strive for rather than the reality. Any concerned adult can help a child in some way: for example, by fighting for children's rights or volunteering for a program that benefits a child. There are many adults who contribute their time, energy, and money to help children, but there is always room for more people who want to aid kids. Every adult can help simply by recognizing the risks a child faces at any given age and then knowing how to protect children from getting into situations where their well-being is endangered. Therefore, this book will explore how parents and concerned adults can help children in a very direct way to prevent these tragedies and deaths before they occur. I will also examine how parents and others can further the cause of children by using their clout to develop community-based programs that work to prevent these unnecessary deaths. New social and political initiatives are urgently needed because governments at all levels have cut back on funds for many programs that directly benefit children, and this has had an effect on the availability of money to aid all types of children's causes and organizations.

In an effort to provide the most up-to-date information, I have researched the current available literature. The data for 1987 on child mortality are the most recent available and were published in their entirety in 1990; the figures must be read and interpreted with this in mind. Though the methods for reporting and recording data vary from area to area and state to state, the conclusions that can be drawn are unmistakable and compelling.

Some readers may wonder why I have chosen to divide "childhood" into three age groups: birth to one year; one year to approximately fourteen years, eleven months; and fifteen to nineteen years, eleven months. Each of these age groups confronts a corresponding distinct set of risks and causes of death. For example, under one year of age, the mortality rate is in general much higher than it is for any other age group, and the corresponding causes of death are distinctly different for infants within that first year. The causes of death from age one to fourteen years, eleven months are very similar and are therefore grouped together. In like manner, children aged fifteen to nineteen years, eleven months die in ways very distinct from those that claim one to fourteen-year-olds or infants. Although there is some overlap in terms of causes of death, these three groups do exhibit diverse mortality statistics and the ranking of the causes of death are different among them.

For instance, suicide is probably the second leading cause of death in fifteen- to nineteen-year-olds, but it is not a leading cause of death in infants or in children between one and fourteen years of age. Self-inflicted death does occur in these younger children, but the results are not as dramatic or evident as in the fifteen- to nineteen-year-old age group. The task of discussing prevalent death statistics is admittedly complex, but I have tried to make the causes within each category as clear as possible. For clarity, I have focused on similarities among groups. When similarities do not exist, I attempt to explain why.

Throughout the text, I remind the reader of the age group I am addressing. However, to facilitate discussion of statistics, I refer to children under one year as "infants," children aged one to fourteen as "children," and fifteen- to nineteen-year-olds as "teens."

The trends and statistics referred to are based on national data collected by the National Center for Health Statistics.* I have analyzed these data and organized them to fit the discussion. Therefore, the reader should bear in mind that my presentation represents my best effort to consolidate very complex data in a more digestible form. Since the most recent data available are from 1987, actual numbers have changed somewhat in the time between data collection and reporting. But the long-term underlying patterns remain the same.

To avoid the risk of overwhelming the reader with statistics, I have concentrated on major causes of death rather than presenting an exhaustive list of every cause within a given category. I have attempted to decipher the major trends in childhood deaths throughout each age continuum. Trends help to determine those situations that need our immediate attention. Since a trend is a dynamic process, causes of death may change over time. A decade from now statistics might highlight entirely different priorities. By the same token, fifteen years ago, no one would have mentioned Acquired Immune Deficiency Syndrome (AIDS). As we face the 1990s, the situation has vastly changed and AIDS has become a priority. Hence, the most prevalent causes of childhood mortality today must be the focus of our efforts. By examining these causes, we take the first step toward finding solutions.

---

*All references to this center for data collection will be prefaced by the acronym NCHS.

Acknowledgments

I would like to thank all those who worked hard to provide me with data as well as support for this project: to my friend and colleague, Joan, who gave me such insight into the African-American community; my children, who respected this work and did the little extras around the house; to my husband, Gary, who read the manuscript in its various forms; and to my typist, Pat Brock-Eisenstein, for her hard work. I also wish to thank all those I interviewed who gave me firsthand insight into the problems confronting our children.

Part One

How Children Die

1

Why Children Die in Our Society

INTRODUCTION

In my days as a practicing nurse, I recall that one of my most demanding roles was helping to give emotional support to the parents of a dying child. Unfortunately, there were many times when I sat with the parents after a treatment had failed to save their "baby." I would try to comfort them as they struggled to find answers: Why had this happened? Their grief and sense of loss were often so overwhelming that few words of mine could soften the ultimate sadness of the moment. On many occasions—more than I care to remember—during my efforts to console them, I would realize that I was crying, too. Even though it wasn't my child, I felt the burden of that grief. Every time I faced another heartbroken couple, I hoped I would never have to experience or share those emotions with any more parents. The fact is that the frequency of such experiences doesn't make it any easier to deal with childhood deaths. As I write this book, I feel the need to remember those moments when I shared someone else's grief and loss. As I begin this discussion of how children die in America, I want readers to realize that the moments I experienced with grieving parents happened all too frequently. I want to convey that, although I review statistics in this presentation, I am well aware that they represent real children and not mere numbers. When I read accounts of children senselessly dying in our nation, I remember the pain and suffering of every one of the children in my care. As a society, we experience some sense of loss when children die. I hope this sensitivity will generate a deeper awareness and thereby spur us to greater efforts at fostering the health, safety, and welfare of our children. By becoming aware of the reasons children die, we may be able to find solutions that work. Sometimes the reasons for childhood death are quite evident, while at other times more research will be needed to find the answers. It is never an easy task, but it is a necessary one if we are to save innocent lives and safeguard our young people.

It is always easier to contemplate cold statistics rather than confront the death of children we have touched and cared for. As adult members of society, we must always remember that these numbers and statistics reflect the senseless destruction of young lives.

SOME FACTS AND NUMBERS

The United States ranks eighteenth among the advanced, industrialized nations of the world in terms of infant mortality. Similar grim statistics can be found in every age group of children. In our country today:

- Each year approximately 40,000 babies die in the first twelve months of life.

- Of all newborns, 6.8 percent suffer from low birth weight (less than 5.5 pounds); 16 percent of all low-birth-weight babies are severely handicapped.

- Congenital defects in newborns, which are detectable by screening, go undetected, resulting in death or mental retardation (4,500 cases annually). (Congenital defects are a leading cause of death in babies less than twenty-eight days old.)

- Of women in their childbearing years (fifteen to forty-four years of age) 9.3 million lack coverage for medical expenses; poor, minority, and unmarried women are overrepresented among the uninsured.

- In 1986, 1,200 deaths were directly related to child abuse (there were 24,000 injuries). There were over one million reports of child abuse in 1983.

- The most common perpetrators of child abuse are the parents.

- In 1985 alone, 1.9 million cases of abuse or neglect were reported.

- Accidents are the leading cause of childhood death in most age groups beyond infancy. This includes vehicular accidents as well as falls, drownings, death by fire, etc. Each year more than 15 million children are injured seriously enough to require medical treatment.

- From 1979 to 1982 motor vehicle accidents were the second leading cause of death in children under one year of age and the leading cause of all deaths in young people aged one to nineteen years. Motor vehicle accidents account for one out of five deaths in children aged one to fourteen years.

- Two out of every five deaths in adolescents are related to motor vehicle accidents—62 percent of tested drivers aged sixteen to nineteen had positive blood-alcohol levels.

- Vital-statistics reports from many urban settings now rank homicide as the third leading cause of death in teenagers.

- The most frequent perpetrators of teenage homicide are acquaintances.

- Causes of teen violence resulting in homicide are most often related to drugs, alcohol, or gang-type activities.

- In 1983, over two hundred children between five and fourteen years of age committed suicide. This accounted for 2.1 percent of deaths in this age group in that year. A 13 percent increase in suicide for this age group is projected by the year 2000.

- Suicide accounts for about 12 percent of all deaths in teenagers. There is a 94 percent increase in suicides projected for fifteen- to nineteen-year-olds by the year 2000.

- For every death by drowning there are at least three by suicide. For every three homicides in the United States there are four suicides. For every two deaths resulting from automobile accidents one young person somewhere commits suicide. Suicide is the second or third highest cause of death among college students (Child Welfare League, 1986; Johnson and Maile, 1987; McIntire and Angle, 1980; Meier, 1985; Miller et al., 1986; NCHS, 1990; *Morbidity and Mortality Weekly Report* [MMWR], July 6, 1990).

PRELIMINARY ANALYSES

These statistics demonstrate that the major threats to infant children are low birth weight and complications related to premature delivery as well as lack of medical care for the mother during pregnancy. What these statistics also illustrate is that in most cases the deaths were probably preventable. Diseases and congenital conditions diagnosed at birth remain major causes of death during the first twenty-eight days of life (NCHS, 1990). Even in the case of illness or disease the vast majority of such deaths were preventable. One research group indicated that in their study more than 70 percent of all deaths reported for infants (i.e., infections acquired after the newborn had been taken home) were clearly preventable. These infants died in circumstances where a parent or health-care worker could have done something to alter the outcome (Druschel and Hale, 1987).

Injury from accidents and violence are also primary causes of death among children one to fourteen years of age in the United States. In fact, motor vehicle injuries, fires, drownings, and homicides were the leading external causes of death at ages one to four years and five to nine years, accounting for nearly 80 percent of all deaths from such causes. Demographic differentials included in this research demonstrate that race is a major factor that must be considered when reviewing these deaths. For example, proportionately more African-American children die from fires and homicides than do white children. Deaths resulting from these external causes accounted for more than two-fifths of the deaths in African-American children aged one to four (Fingerhut et al., 1988). As with infants, the majority of these deaths were preventable with some type of adult or legal intervention. In terms of sex differences, 65 percent of the deaths in males were due to external causes in this age group. Specifically, pedestrian-related motor vehicle accidents and drownings account for the largest proportion of deaths in one- to fourteen-year-old males (Fingerhut et al., 1988).

Congenital anomalies and cancer are leading internal causes of death in children from one to fourteen years of age. Some of these conditions are preventable or treatable.

In our teen population (fifteen to nineteen years of age), accidents, homicides, and suicides are leading causes of death. As with the other age groups, these types of death are entirely preventable. Unfortunately, these trends may change very little in the years to come. Teens seem especially vulnerable to unnecessary external causes of death. Research targeting this population to gain greater insight into their behaviors and experiences illustrates their vulnerability and how truly at risk they are. A National Adolescent Study Health Survey (NASHS) was conducted in 1987. It was the first survey since the 1960s to look at teenage health behavior and the risk factors associated with teen death, and is therefore especially germane to our discussions of child mortality. The survey addressed health-related topics for which no data base exists: unintentional injuries; fighting and violence; suicide; use of tobacco, alcohol, and drugs; and other aspects of health behavior. The survey included eighth and tenth graders.

We already know that accidents are the leading cause of death in teens fifteen to nineteen years old, and two out of every five of these deaths involve motor vehicles. Over half (62 percent) of the vehicular accidents involve alcohol abuse by the teenage driver and passengers. From the NASHS survey (Miller et al., 1986), it is reported that 56 percent of the students do not wear seat belts when they drive or ride in a car, and 44 percent of the tenth graders and 32 percent of the eighth graders had ridden in a car with a driver who had used drugs and/or alcohol within a month prior to the survey (MMWR, March 10, 1989).

Homicide and violence are also leading causes of death in teenagers. Some cities rank homicide as the second or third leading cause of death among teens in this age category. According to the NASHS, 49 percent of the boys and 28 percent of the girls surveyed reported having at least one physical fight during the past year. Four percent of those surveyed reported being threatened and 23 percent of the boys said they carried a knife at least once during the past year. Three percent of the boys reported taking a handgun to school in the year prior to the survey (MMWR, March 10, 1990).

In terms of suicide, 25 percent of the boys and 42 percent of the girls reported that they had at some time during their lives seriously considered committing suicide. Eighteen percent of the females and 11 percent of the males had actually attempted to hurt themselves in a way that could have resulted in their death (MMWR, March 10, 1989). This is evidence that the behavior of teens continues to place many of them in a high-risk category. Therefore, these statistics reinforce the belief that little will change in the years to come.

SUMMARY

Tables 1 and 2 reflect a breakdown of the causes of death in children over the age of one year. Infant mortality will be dealt with in detail in chapter 2.

From this brief overview, we can proceed to a more in-depth discussion of how our children die. If we are going to combat childhood death, we must be aware of the primary causes of these casualties. This is no easy task since the primary causes of death in children vary according to their chronological age, race or ethnic background, geographic location, and a variety of other demographic factors.

TABLE 1. MAJOR CAUSES OF DEATH IN CHILDREN AGED ONE TO FOURTEEN YEARS
(Rank Ordered; Total Deaths = 16,216; NCHS, 1990)

1. Accidents

   A. Motor vehicle-related accidents:

      (1) riding as a passenger in a car/vehicle

      (2) pedestrian

      (3) cyclist

   B. Nonvehicular accidents involving:

   CAUSES

One to Four Years	Five to Fourteen Years
(1) fires	(1) drowning
(2) drowning	(2) fires
(3) inhalation/ingestion of foreign objects	(3) handguns and firearms
(4) falls	(4) falls
(5) poisonings/ingestion of foreign substances	(5) poisonings/ingestion of foreign substances

2. Neoplasms (Cancer)

   A. Malignant neoplasms of lymphatic and hematopoietic tissues

   B. Malignant neoplasms of body structures

      1. various organs

      2. brain

      3. bone, connective tissue

3. Congenital anomalies manifested as:

   A. Anomalies of the heart and circulatory system

   B. Anomalies of the nervous system

4. Diseases/disorders of the nervous system

5. Diseases/disorders of the cardiovascular system

6. Homicide

7. Diseases/disorders of the respiratory system

TABLE 2. MAJOR CAUSES OF DEATH IN TEENS
AGED FIFTEEN TO NINETEEN YEARS
(Rank Ordered)

1. Accidents:

   A. Motor vehicle-related accidents:

      (1) driver of motor vehicle

      (2) passenger in motor vehicle

      (3) motorcyclist (driver/passenger)

      (4) pedestrian

      (5) bicyclist

   B. Nonvehicular accidents involving:

      (1) drowning

      (2) falls

      (3) poisonings/ingestion of foreign substances

      (4) handguns and firearms

2. Suicide by the following methods:

   A. Guns/Firearms

   B. Hanging

   C. Ingestion of Substances

      (1) pain-killers

      (2) aspirin

3. Homicide. Assault with:

   A. Gun/Firearm

   B. Knife/Sharp Object

   C. Unspecified

2

Infant Death

INTRODUCTION

The death rate in the first year of life is so high that it warrants being examined separately. The infant mortality rate is generally regarded as a quality-of-life indicator for both the health and the welfare of a population (Miller et al., 1986). It is a combination of specific statistics that takes into consideration the number of infants who die in the first twenty-eight days of life (neonatal death rate) plus the number of deaths attributed to infants from twenty-eight days to one year of age (postneonatal death rate). These rates are calculated per one thousand live births. As indicated previously, mortality in the first twenty-eight days of life tends to be associated with low birth weight and with factors occurring prenatally (during pregnancy), during birth, and in the first weeks of life. This low birth weight occurs as a consequence of various environmental factors, including poor maternal nutrition and health practices, lack of quality care during pregnancy and delivery, and congenital defects not compatible with physically sustaining life. Mortality beyond the first twenty-eight days of life is linked to inadequate nutrition or sanitation, unsafe living conditions, and the lack of access to health-care services (Miller et al., 1986). For instance, the death rate from falls for children under age one is higher than it is for any other age group, reflecting that the safety of a baby's living conditions is a significant contributing factor in a number of infant deaths in this age group. Also, the number of infectious diseases that result in death escalates after the first twenty-eight days, which of course is related to the sanitary conditions surrounding the infant.

24

What are the consequences of these factors? In 1983, 40,627 infants died before their first birthday (Miller et al., 1986). In 1987, 38,408 infants died (NCHS, 1990). The United States ranked eighteenth in infant mortality in the world (Miller et al., 1986), which means that seventeen other countries did a better job at protecting their infants from death than we did. Spain, Ireland, Japan, Germany, and France, among others, are ahead of us in safeguarding the lives of their infants (Children's Defense Fund, 1989). This reflects how far we have fallen behind the other leading industrialized nations in preventing infant death in the first year of life. Nonwhite infants in this country die at almost twice the rate of white infants and the disparity continues to escalate. Death occurring in the first twenty-eight days of life accounts for nearly two-thirds of all infant deaths, with the largest portion of these deaths occurring in the first week of life.

The Department of Health and Human Services, in its objectives for the nation's health, declared that by 1990 the United States would reach an infant death rate of only nine per thousand live births; that no racial or ethnic group would have an infant mortality rate in excess of 12 deaths per thousand live births; and that the newborn death rate would be no higher than 6.5 deaths per thousand births (Miller et al., 1986). However, there are still 22 states that have an infant mortality rate above 9 per thousand live births and over 43 states that have mortality rates above 12 per thousand live births for nonwhite infants (NCHS, 1990). Although the methods for recording, reporting, and retrieving these data may not be as accurate or timely as we would like (sometimes three to four years later), this information does reflect the fact that many areas in our country, for a variety of reasons, have not succeeded in accomplishing these 1990 objectives with regard to infant mortality.

The U.S. Public Health Service has now issued a set of 339 proposed objectives for the year 2000. Compared with the 1990 goals, the new objectives reflect a greater emphasis on prevention of disability through screening and by paying closer attention to high-risk groups. These goals include an infant mortality of no more than seven deaths per thousand life births (MMWR, September 22, 1989). Until the age of one year, the death rate for these infants is as high as it is for mature adults sixty-five years of age and older. Approximately nine to eighteen babies out of every thousand will die before their first birthday if past and present statistics persist.

CAUSES OF INFANT MORTALITY: GENERAL OVERVIEW

Because the reasons infants die are quite different from those that explain the death of children over one year of age, we will examine infant fatalities separately.

As was outlined earlier, the infant mortality rate is divided into two periods: the neonatal period—those deaths occurring in the first twenty-eight days of life; and the postneonatal period—those occurring from twenty-eight days to the age of approximately one year. The National Center for Health Statistics (NCHS) has compiled a list of causes and rank-ordered them by how frequently they occur per one thousand live births. The center then combines the deaths from these two periods and rank orders an overall list for the first year of life. We will look at both the neonatal and post-neonatal periods separately and then examine the combined list. These statistics describe tabulations for the year 1987.

As we discussed previously, the tabulation of data is usually several years behind. However, these are the most current data available as we go to press. In reviewing the data from 1979 to 1987, the causes of death and their frequency seem fairly stable. In other words, the variation in terms of their rank order changes little. Therefore, we can assume that these statistics for years since 1987 will be very similar to that year.

The Neonatal Period

During the first twenty-eight days of life, the leading cause of death was congenital anomalies (5,740 deaths). These are birth defects that occur from some disturbance or abnormal change during the baby's development while in the mother's womb. There are malformations or defects in the developing infant's physical structure that, upon birth and separation from the mother, are incompatible with life. The vast majority of these death-producing birth defects are associated with an abnormality of the physical structure in the heart, the circulatory system, or the respiratory system (NCHS, 1990). Other defects caused by genetic abnormalities may be so severe that they, too, cause death before or during delivery.

The second leading cause of death in this neonatal period is disorders related to premature delivery and low birth weight (3,303 deaths). This prematurity and low birth weight in most instances can be related to lack of prenatal care resulting from economic barriers and lack of access to health care, and sometimes to the unhealthy lifestyle of the pregnant mother

(Children's Defense Fund, 1989).* It has also been reported that the ocrence of low birth weight is related to a pregnant mother's marital status. Unmarried motherhood was associated with an overall elevated infant mortality rate, especially in the prenatal period (MMWR, August 3, 1990). It is important to note that the neonatal death rate for African-American babies is roughly double that for white children.

The third leading cause of death in neonates is *respiratory distress syndrome* (NCHS, 1990), which is produced by a variety of factors associated with an underdeveloped respiratory system that fails to function properly. We will discuss this in more depth in the section on diseases in children (chapter 4). This complex set of symptoms is responsible for 3,086 deaths in the early days of life.

Complications both during pregnancy and during the delivery are the fourth and fifth leading causes of neonatal death. Combined they were the cause of over two thousand infant deaths in 1987 (NCHS, 1990). Infections that occur during pregnancy and trauma associated with labor and/ or delivery are responsible for additional infant deaths (821). These rank six, nine, and ten respectively.

Sudden Infant Death Syndrome (SIDS) in the first twenty-eight days of life accounts for about 2 percent of the neonatal death rate, while pneumonia and influenza still produce over 150 deaths per year.

In addition to the above causes of death, which are directly related to problems during pregnancy, labor, and/or delivery, accidents and their adverse affects as well as homicides rank fourteenth and fifteenth for this age group.

The Postneonatal Period

In the postneonatal period the leading cause of death is Sudden Infant Death Syndrome (NCHS, 1990), which results in over 4,500 deaths in children from twenty-eight days to one year of age. Congenital anomalies (birth defects) rank second, and again the defects associated with the heart, circulatory, and respiratory structures appear to be the most lethal.

Accidents, which ranked relatively low in the neonatal period (fourteenth), rank third in the postneonatal age group, while homicide moves into the sixth position. These causes of death will be discussed in more detail later in this chapter.

---

*This should not be construed as a value judgment but rather an objective assessment of the mother's willingness to take proper care to safeguard the child.

Various types of infections seem to be particularly prevalent factors relating to the high death rate in the postneonatal period. Infections such as meningitis (inflammation of the layers of tissue covering the brain), bronchitis (inflammation of the lungs), and other bacterial and viral illnesses seem to occur more frequently in this age group than in neonates.

INFANCY: A SUMMARY OF STATISTICS

Listed below in Table 3 is a rank-ordering of the leading causes of infant death when the neonatal and postneonatal periods are combined. As can be seen, the rank-ordering of causes is very different. The period termed "infancy" (0 to 1 year of age) is probably the most difficult to analyze since the causes of death change over a relatively short period of time. Therefore, when discussing infant mortality, it is essential that we address the differences between the neonatal and postneonatal periods so that all the facts associated with the death rate are fully understood.

TABLE 3. LEADING CAUSES OF INFANT, NEONATAL, AND POSTNEONATAL DEATH: UNITED STATES: 1987
(Each Period Rank Ordered)

INFANT (Overall cause of death for both neonatal and postneonatal periods)

1. congenital anomalies (defects)
2. Sudden Infant Death Syndrome (SIDS)
3. disorders relating to short gestation and unspecified low birth weight
4. respiratory distress syndrome
5. newborn affected by maternal complications of pregnancy
6. accidents and adverse effects
7. infections specific to the perinatal*
8. newborn affected by complications of placenta, cord, and membranes
9. intrauterine hypoxia†and birth asphyxia‡

---

*Referring to period just prior, during, or after birth.
†Inadequate oxygen in the lungs and blood.
‡Suffocation.

10. pneumonia and influenza
11. neonatal hemorrhage
12. homicide
13. septicemia*
14. birth trauma
15. meningitis†

NEONATAL (0 to 28 days of age)

1. congenital anomalies
2. disorders relating to short gestation and unspecified low birth weight
3. respiratory distress syndrome
4. newborn affected by maternal complications of pregnancy
5. newborn affected by complications of placenta, cord, and membranes
6. infections specific to the perinatal period
7. intrauterine hypoxia and birth asphyxia
8. Sudden Infant Death Syndrome (SIDS)
9. neonatal hemorrhage
10. birth trauma
11. pneumonia and influenza
12. newborn affected by maternal conditions that may be unrelated to present pregnancy
13. newborn affected by other complications of labor and delivery
14. accidents and adverse effects
15. homicide

POSTNEONATAL (28 days to 1 year of age)

1. Sudden Infant Death Syndrome (SIDS)
2. congenital anomalies
3. accidents and adverse effects
4. pneumonia and influenza
5. septicemia
6. homicide
7. respiratory distress syndrome

---

*Condition caused by bacteria in the blood stream.
†Inflammation of membranes surrounding the brain and spinal cord.

8. meningitis
9. bronchitis and bronchiolitis
10. malignant neoplasms, including neoplasms of lymphatic and hematopoietic tissues
11. gastritis, duodenitis, and noninfective enteritis and colitis
12. viral diseases
13. meningococcal infection
14. intrauterine hypoxia and birth asphyxia
15. hernia of abdominal cavity and intestinal obstruction without mention of hernia

REASONS FOR INFANT DEATH

Lack of Prenatal Care

Many factors affect the birth of a baby, and some of them begin well before the infant is even delivered. Children in the United States often receive a death sentence at the moment of conception. The major reasons infants die at birth and in the first year of life are premature delivery, birth defects, and low birth weight (NCHS, 1990). Low birth weight means the infant weighs less than what has been termed "normal" (five and one-half pounds). In fact, two-thirds of these infants' deaths occur in the first week of life. One might assume that low birth weight and congenital anomalies are not preventable because they result from what happens to the baby as it develops in the womb. However, these abnormalities can often be tied to how the mother cares for herself while she is pregnant.

Many babies in this country are born to mothers who do not get adequate prenatal care prior to giving birth. A major portion of these new mothers are just children themselves, teenagers who do not have an opportunity to see to their own health care, let alone their developing unborn child's. Other expectant mothers may be too poor or too ignorant about the necessity of medical attention and its availability during pregnancy to get the kind of care they need before delivery. There are many reports showing that a major portion of the low-birth-weight problem is related to factors that stem from poverty, lack of education, or access to adequate health-care services (Miller et al., 1986).

Low birth weight is also related to race or ethnic group. The death rate resulting from low birth weight in African-American infants is proportionately higher than it is for Caucasian infants (Miller et al., 1986;

NCHS, 1990). Hispanic women in the United States are at even greater risk than African-Americans of receiving inadequate care and delivering low-birth-weight babies (Miller et al., 1986). Therefore, although the weight problem resulting from sporadic or the complete absence of care during pregnancy is a major factor in the death of white infants, it is a considerably greater one in the death of African-American and Hispanic infants.

The Institute of Medicine (IOM) reports research evidence indicating that low birth weight is directly related to lack of prenatal care. The institute lists six major barriers to the utilization of prenatal services by U.S. women:

1. financial constraints

2. limited availability of maternal-care providers, especially for the disadvantaged

3. insufficient prenatal services at sites used by high-risk women

4. experiences, attitudes, and beliefs among women that discourage seeking prenatal care

5. inadequate transportation and child-care services

6. inadequate recruitment of hard-to-reach populations (IOM, 1985).

High-risk women tend to be teenagers, unmarried, and nonwhite (Miller et al., 1986; MMWR, August 3, 1990).

Besides lack of prenatal care, there are other problems society must deal with that may also produce premature or low-birth-weight babies: for example, drug and alcohol addiction in the mother, poor nutrition, smoking, or sexually transmitted diseases that are not treated effectively before pregnancy. Many of the congenital abnormalities and genetic anomalies found in this age group can be lethal and may ultimately be tied to the mother's negative health habits and to her lack of medical care during pregnancy.

The complications associated with pregnancy, labor, and delivery are often very manageable and foreseeable with adequate medical care. However, for a variety of reasons, many pregnant women do not get the medical care they need. By the time they deliver the child, it is too late for successful intervention.

Not long ago, I had occasion to talk to a pregnant African-American teenager. She was fourteen years old, six-months pregnant, and her mother had basically told her she was "on her own." This young woman had not yet seen a doctor. After her mother's rejection, she was afraid to approach anyone else for help. She felt that people would "look down on her." Consequently, she was six-months pregnant and had not seen a physician. Although she had access to medical help, she was afraid to tap this resource. She hid her pregnancy as long as possible but suddenly delivered twins prematurely. One infant died at birth; the other has shown signs of mental retardation. She would not agree to seek medical care until she was in the final throes of labor. Consequently, she had a very difficult delivery because one baby was in the breech position,* and this was not dealt with until it was too late. If she had had a physician involved during her pregnancy, the outcome would probably have been much improved.

One study has shown that the ramifications of poverty alone negatively influence birth outcomes and increase the incidence of infant death (Stockwell and Swanson, 1988). Sometimes, it is apparent that even when help is available, women will avoid medical care for a variety of reasons. These may be related to their age, culture, and economic situation (Miller et al., 1986). Recent research indicates that even in areas with virtually universal access to high-tech medical care, the rate of death for African-American infants is much higher than for whites (Miller et al., 1986).

Sexually Transmitted Diseases

One factor that affects our unborn babies concerns the various side effects of diseases spread by sexual contact. A mother who has a venereal disease can pass the disease on to her unborn child during pregnancy. This further contributes to the number of babies with low birth weight and those delivered prematurely. Many sexually transmitted diseases (syphilis, gonorrhea, etc.) have existed throughout history. However, there are others that have recently become even more threatening. One of the major concerns today is, of course, Acquired Immune Deficiency Syndrome (AIDS). This disease can also be transmitted from mother to child during pregnancy. Even more problematic is that it can be spread by the sharing of needles among addicts, in addition to direct sexual contact. Not only do sexually transmitted diseases contribute to the increase of low-birth-weight babies, but they also produce birth defects that may cause other conditions that kill children immediately at birth or later in infancy, or render them disabled. Congenital anomalies continue to be a major cause of infant death.

---

*The fetus was emerging from the uterus feet first.

In the case of AIDS, pregnancy has become a mechanism to infect a whole new generation. In fact, in 1988 there were 447 cases of prenatal transmission (MMWR, March 17, 1989). This disease is an epidemic threatening all segments of society including our unborn children; the problem may be getting worse and it appears that the numbers of babies born to mothers with AIDS will increase dramatically in the next ten years since the number of women infected is also growing. The same can be said of all sexually transmitted diseases.

The simple truth is that many babies could be saved if we took better care of pregnant mothers. We need to make sure that these mothers get good, readily available care and that they are educated about how sexually transmitted diseases can cause birth defects, other long-term health problems, and even death.

Drugs, Alcohol, and Infant Death

Mothers addicted to various substances have a much greater risk of producing low-birth-weight babies. These addictions may also produce side effects or birth defects that can result in death at birth or later in infancy. A pregnant mother who is addicted to alcohol or drugs passes that addiction on to her developing infant. At birth the infant has to deal with the same physiological problems of addiction and withdrawal as the mother does when she is cut off from her supply of alcohol or drugs. In addition, these mothers often do not attempt to obtain good care during their pregnancy, which further reduces the infant's chances of survival. Although many hospitals are proficient in the treatment of infants born to mothers who are drug addicts or alcoholics, the side effects in the infant may be too far advanced and the physical damage too great for this help to be successful. The odds are slim that the infant will overcome this hurdle: in fact, the survival rate is disappointing. Low-birth-weight infants have enough difficulty surviving without being burdened with added problems. Being born to an addicted mother makes the odds of survival even less.

Drug and alcohol addiction is a major concern in this country; all too often the consequences of these addictions are passed on to our children, even before birth. It is also well documented that certain drugs, like cocaine, have negative consequences for fetal circulation (van de Bor et al., 1990). I recently talked to a friend who works as a maternal-child nurse in a local prenatal clinic in an inner city location. She told me that about one-third of the mothers who enter the clinic are addicted to various kinds or combinations of drugs. She and her coworkers try hard to wean these mothers off all drugs, but they must often remain content to narrow the addiction down to just one drug. Then their pregnant patients are easier to treat. This nurse also expressed concern for the babies who survive. The children of cocaine-addicted mothers often suffer from behavioral and physical aberrations that make them extremely difficult to raise and nurture.

Nutrition

The impact of poor nutrition on low birth weight should not be under-estimated. A pregnant woman who lacks an adequate diet may produce a child with low birth weight or other ailments. Poor nutrition can hamper the development of the fetus in utero. Mothers may neglect to eat the proper foods because of poverty, general neglect of their own health, ignor-ance, or addiction. The problem was so pervasive in this country that the federal government instituted the WIC (Women, Infants, and Children Supplemental Food) Program. However, only about 40 percent of the women entitled to its benefits take advantage of them (Children's Defense Fund, 1989). If we can improve the mother's nutritional status, we can improve the baby's chances of survival.

Stress

Several studies have suggested that psychosocial factors such as stress, anxiety, and poor social support systems may affect the outcome of preg-nancy. A poor outcome was defined as low birth weight or neonatal death. There is reason to believe that severe stress in the final two trimesters (the last six months) of pregnancy can be related to serious complications and infant mortality (Williamson et al., 1989).

Smoking and Low Birth Weight

It has become a well-known fact in the late 1980s that smoking has a direct impact on the weight of a pregnant mother's unborn child (Servonsky and Opas, 1987). Therefore, although smoking previously has been an accepted norm in our culture, it has recently been attacked because of its negative health consequences and its connection with the incidence of low birth weight.

Firsthand Knowledge

Many of the social and medical problems I have just discussed in abstract terms became immediate and personal when I met a young woman— I'll call her Millie—who had been sexually abused as a child and had left home at the early age of thirteen. Overcoming the odds, she had managed to finish most of her high school education. Millie had lived all over the city—in shelters, with friends, and on the streets. By her own admission, she had survived with the help of friends, financial aid, and, on occasion, stealing food and clothing. Millie did not take drugs on a regular basis but said she occasionally used "pot" and "cocaine." During our acquaintance, she confided that she was four months pregnant and had not seen a physician to that point. Millie had taken drugs early in her pregnancy; she was almost three months pregnant before realizing that she was expecting a child. Millie did not have an ongoing relationship with the prospective father and knew little about his background. She had not used any means of birth control prior to the pregnancy and she had been sexually active for the three years she had been on the street.

Millie wanted her baby and had not considered abortion at any point; she realized she had to have some means of supporting herself and her child. I was very concerned for her welfare, directed her to medical care, and tried to assist her in finding more permanent living arrangements. She was very suspicious and reluctant to accept help from me or any other adult. Eventually, she did get medical help in the fifth month of her pregnancy but delivered prematurely a month later. The child died at birth. I was struck by the fact that there were two casualties here— this beautiful young woman who had been abused by her parents and then neglected by society, and her unborn child. This child was conceived in ignorance and nurtured with neglect. It wasn't just her child; it was ours as well. "Children having children" is a frequent public lament these days, but the heart-wrenching reality doesn't always hit home as poignantly as it should. Pregnancy in young American teenage women continues at an alarming rate.

IMPLICATIONS

Unfortunately, our society has moved very slowly in finding workable solutions to the problem of teen pregnancy. Somehow, we need to reach our teenagers, without making moral judgments about pregnancy or the available alternatives. Once they are pregnant and have made certain choices, we are obligated to protect the unborn child as well as the welfare of the mother. Birth control to prevent these unplanned pregnancies appears to be a possible solution. However, many young women do not use any means of contraceptive prevention or protection. They lack the necessary education and preparation with regard to birth control. Perhaps these young women are not comfortable seeking help or are not mature enough or informed enough once they do become pregnant. I was amazed at how much my young acquaintance expected her child to brighten her already hard life and equally amazed that she knew very little about how to protect the developing child she so desperately wanted. Low-birth-weight babies, infants with birth defects, and increasing numbers of infant deaths will continue among a large sector of our nation's young women unless we find a way to reach out and help them understand the need for good care during pregnancy, and if need be, provide it to them. It would be great if birth control were the primary solution, but the fact remains that there will be unplanned pregnancies where the young mother decides to continue the pregnancy and keep the child. At that point, we need to ensure that these babies are healthy and normal, and that implies education about a healthy pregnancy and early prenatal care.

Other factors will have to be addressed that contribute to low-birth-weight babies and birth defects, such as drug and alcohol addiction and maternal diseases. These are major and persistent problems that society must address not just for pregnant women but for all its citizens. However, we must begin to find solutions through education and research so that our unborn do not have to pay the ultimate price.

We can educate but we still have to consider the costs, especially in economic terms, of these solutions. The Children's Defense Fund (1989) contends that cost savings can be realized if we provide funds for prenatal care. In fact, for every dollar spent on such care, we save three dollars on health-care that would have been necessary if the pregnancy produced a premature or low-birth-weight baby. Again, if education were the only factor, then we could launch a massive effort to inform women about the importance of taking care of themselves during pregnancy. But realistically, that's not the only solution. The prenatal care these women need must be available at low cost. Statistics show that most low-birth-weight or premature babies are born to poor, unmarried women or to women who lack the financial means or health insurance to pay for good prenatal care. How available are these services to this "at risk" group? If indeed we are "a kinder and gentler nation," shouldn't we address this question?

What choices do poor women have with regard to prenatal care? Are these women doomed to failure under our present system? It is a fact that if we invest in prenatal care, we can save a great deal of money: caring for disabled babies is much more expensive than providing adequate care early on (Children's Defense Fund, 1989).

SUMMARY

One might think that because the United States has such advanced medical care and is one of the most affluent countries in the world, the number of babies born healthy would be statistically high compared to other industrialized nations. But the fact of the matter is we are not even in the top ten, and one of the primary reasons for this is our high infant death rate. We have talked about some of the social (i.e., poverty) and medical problems (i.e., drug or alcohol abuse, etc.) that can result in low birth weight. But the most concrete reason for infant death related to prematurity, low birth weight, and birth defects is the simple lack of adequate education about good health practices and the lack of good care and treatment of problems during pregnancy.

In order to prevent infant death we must be aware of why it happens. It's hard to ignore the facts. Premature, low-birth-weight babies most often are the children of young women without any support, financial or otherwise. Our society is not reaching these women, and until we do our infant death rate will reflect our failure in this regard. We also need to examine why more African-American and Hispanic babies die at birth than Caucasian babies. Most of the facts are in, now "it's our move."

CONCLUSIONS ON INFANT DEATH

In reviewing the infant death rate, it is clear that certain general factors are pertinent. First, it is apparent that at least nine of our fifty states have an infant mortality rate that exceeds nine per one thousand live births. Of twenty-eight states with more than twenty-five hundred African-American births, twenty-one have infant mortality rates that exceed two per one thousand births (Miller et al., 1990). Second, it is also apparent that there have been dramatic decreases in this mortality rate over the past seventy-five years. This reduction demonstrates the impact of improved medical care and technological advances in neonatal life-support systems.

In 1915, for example, the rate of infant mortality was 95.7 per 1,000 live births, whereas today it is 10.1. However, it is equally important to note that the mortality rate for African-American infants in 1987 was twice that of white infants (17.9 versus 8.6). This, too, seems to be a persistent pattern when looking at the mortality rates for individual states (NCHS, 1990). So even though advances in medical care have had a dramatic positive impact on reducing the overall number of deaths among infants, it is not having the same impact on African-American children aged zero months to one year.

In reviewing these statistics, it is noteworthy that the highest frequency of infant death occurs in the first seven days of life. Of the 38,408 infants who died in 1987, statistics show 20,471 died less than seven days after birth. By day twenty-eight, this number increased to 24,627, demonstrating the significant risk to infant survival during the first twenty-seven days. Of the 24,627 who died in early infancy, 13,872 were male children and 10,755 were female. When racial differences are examined, it is apparent that male children of whatever race have a higher death rate than female infants, and as previously discussed, African-American infants of both sexes have a mortality rate roughly twice that of white infants of both sexes (NCHS, 1990). In conclusion, the top three causes of infant death are related to internal causes associated with fetal development during pregnancy. Since this is such a pervasive problem, I have devoted this chapter to it.

3

Accidents

INTRODUCTION

Accidents are probably the most unsettling cause of death in infants and in children of every age because they seem so easily preventable. Every year, automobile-related accidents, drownings, fires, and falls claim many young lives. While talking with a group of young mothers at a social gathering, I asked what they thought were the most common causes of death in children the same age as their own—one year. Though most of the mothers were very aware of the types of accidents that threatened their children, each of these predominantly well-educated, prosperous, and devoted parents admitted that at least one of her children had experienced an accidental injury in which medical treatment was required.

One mother said that her child had fallen down the stairs while she was at home doing laundry. When the woman's back was turned, her daughter had crawled to the stairs and pulled herself up several steps and then fell backward onto the floor below. As a result of this experience, the woman bought a safety gate and now confines her little girl to a safe space close by when she is busy doing something around the house. This mother was lucky. As table 3 in chapter 2 clearly shows, falls are a frequent cause of death in children under one year of age; most injuries to the children of this group of women had come from falls. Securing the youngster in a safe, comfortable space is crucial, especially if the parent has to leave the child, if only for just a few minutes.

Another woman in the group—we'll call her Alice—had a child who drank a bottle of nail polish remover. This resulted in a trip to the emergency room. The child was saved because Alice reacted immediately. However, if she had not reached her child in time, Alice may not have been quite so lucky. Preventing such incidents by placing poisonous substances out of the reach of small children is a far better alternative.

Yet another member of the audience, whom I've named Brenda, had a small child who was seriously burned. As part of her morning ritual, Brenda plugged in the curling iron as she got ready for work. While she was briefly out of the room, it fell off the bureau onto the rug near her active, crawling infant. The curious child picked up the hot iron and held on. Piercing screams brought Brenda running, but the child had already suffered a nasty burn that required treatment.

The point here is that small children need to be protected. None of these incidents produced a fatal injury—this time—but one inattentive moment is all it takes for potentially lethal consequences to befall a curious or playful youngster. None of these accidents would have occurred if the mother had put the child in a playpen or had someone keep watch while she was otherwise occupied. These examples demonstrate how potentially deadly accidents can occur around the home.

In the pages that follow, we will examine the various types of accidents that claim the lives of our children. It is important to note that of all accidents the total number of deaths involving vehicles is roughly equal to the total number of deaths from all other nonvehicular accidents combined.

ACCIDENTS INVOLVING INFANTS

From 1979 to 1982, the second leading cause of death in children under the age of one involved injuries inflicted as a result of motor vehicle accidents (Miller et al., 1986). By 1987, these accidents claimed the lives of more infants aged one year or younger than any other type of accidental death (NCHS, 1990). In recent years, the mandatory use of infant car seats has reduced the number of such deaths related to vehicular collisions. Yet there are still parents who neglect to use infant safety seats. Many insist on holding their children despite legislation requiring that infants be secured in a safety seat at all times. More important, there is ample evidence that these seats do save the lives of infants who are involved in car crashes.

I recall an automobile accident in which a baby was crushed between its mother and the car dashboard. The mother survived the accident with minor injuries; however, the infant died immediately. Even though a safety seat was securely positioned in the back seat of the car, the mother decided to hold the baby while her husband drove the short distance home from a relative's house. It was a choice that cost their baby its life.

The second leading cause of accidental death in this period of infancy from birth to eleven months is obstruction of the respiratory tract and suffocation as a result of inhaling food or ingesting objects that block the windpipe. An obstruction can result not only from bits of food but from toys or small objects that infants place in their mouths during play. A child's airway can also become obstructed by an infection that causes tissues in the throat to swell from inflammation.

A few years ago I was at a family picnic with neighbors, friends, and a number of very small children in attendance. As one often finds at picnics of this sort, there were bowls of nibble-type foods like pretzels and potato chips on all the tables. One nine-month-old child was playing quietly in his playpen, until an older child of about five gave the infant a potato chip. This simply delighted the little fellow as he gladly chomped down on the chip. However, a large piece became lodged in his airway and suddenly he could not breathe. When an object blocks the airway, often a child can neither cry nor make a sound. Luckily, his dilemma became immediately apparent to adults close by: I noticed that the infant was noiselessly gagging and that he was not able to cough effectively to dislodge the object himself. I rushed over, picked him up, and, holding his body and head in a downward position, I delivered four blows to his upper back with the heel of one hand. This successfully dislodged the piece of potato chip. The child immediately began to cry and his skin color dramatically changed from ashen grey to a healthy pink. The effect of removing the obstruction was immediately apparent.

All adults should be familiar with the method developed to aid a choking person. Posters demonstrating how to perform it are publicly displayed in many restaurants. With infants, one initially picks the child up and delivers four blows to the back, followed by chest thrusts, as long as the infant appears conscious (AHA, 1987). If the child is unconscious, one should try to rouse him and ascertain whether or not there is a pulse or respiration. This brief description of the procedures for responding to a very young choking victim is by no means inclusive, and all adults should consult their local Heart Association or American Red Cross to learn how to become proficient in the method. In the above instance the child was saved, but not every incident of choking has a happy ending.

A colleague once told me the story of a young mother of two small children for whom she babysat while attending college. One child was eighteen-months old and the other was about two to three months of age. One afternoon the older child was especially active and wanted to go outside to play. The mother placed the infant in its crib and proceeded to take her older child outside for playtime. When the mother and child returned, her infant was lying in the crib, grey and unresponsive. By the time emergency aid arrived the infant was beyond help. The baby had choked on its own bib string.

A neighbor told me about an incident involving a friend of hers who used a small blanket to prop up a bottle of formula so her baby could drink while she answered the doorbell. The woman stood talking with the visitor and completely forgot the baby with its bottle. The infant in the meantime had vomited the formula, thus blocking its airway. The child choked to death in that short time.

When my own little girl was about ten months old, I was visiting with a neighbor, whose child was playing with clay. The neighbor's older child decided to pack my daughter's nose with clay and give her a little to eat, too. This game almost became lethal for my little girl because she couldn't breathe through her nose and gagged on the piece of clay that had been put in her mouth. I nearly lost my daughter but, thankfully, I was close by, and when I checked on her, I was able to remove the obstruction.

As a nurse, I saw many children enter the emergency room with asthma, sore throats, and other upper respiratory infections. At times, because of the infectious process, the tissue around the airway becomes swollen and inflamed. If the infection is not treated, this tissue can swell so much that it partially or even completely closes the infant's airway. This is a very common cause of airway obstruction in infants; such obstruction, if not reversed, can result in death.

Another frequently occurring form of nonvehicular accidental death is that caused by fire. For those under one year of age, the 1987 statistics (NCHS, 1990) rank smoke, fire, and related situations as the third most common cause of accidental death in infants.

Drowning is another type of accident that is equally preventable during infancy. The danger seems to be especially high for the first twenty-eight days of life (Miller et al., 1986). These drownings may result from adult ignorance of safety precautions or lack of care and supervision while a baby is bathed.

Ranking fifth among the causes of accidental death in children under the age of one year is the broad category of *falls* (NCHS, 1990). There are, according to the National Center for Health Statistics, various classificatons of falls: those occurring between two heights, those on the same level, and a portion termed unspecified. Virtually no deaths resulted from falls occurring on the same level in this age group. The majority of lethal infant falls are those occurring between two varying levels or heights. For infants there are no ostensibly significant differences with respect to gender and race when it comes to the frequency of falls (NCHS, 1990). All infants take tumbles, especially when they are learning to crawl and walk. The most potentially deadly falls occur when a child tumbles from a height to a surface below. Babies have extraordinary agility when getting into dangerous spots but little coordination in terms of getting down from high places safely on their own. I have read newspaper stories describing infants who have crawled out of windows in their home and have fallen to the surface below. As a nurse, I took care of an infant in the hospital after he fell out of an open second floor window of his home. The infant was hospitalized with head trauma for months after the fall, and he sustained severe brain damage. The child ultimately died several months later from complications of that head injury.

My own daughter at seven or eight months learned to pull herself to a standing position in her crib. She would hold onto the crib rail and bounce up and down. Because she was so small, it never occurred to me that she could bounce high enough to go completely over the rail. How wrong I was! One morning, over the rail she went. Luckily, she landed on her backside rather than her head. Never again did I assume anything about her abilities. I put the crib mattress at the lowest position possible and made sure the side rails were up no matter what when she was in her crib.

Based on some useful experiences, I think parents should watch small infants with older siblings. I recall one incident in which a small baby was injured when his three-year-old sister decided to take her infant brother out of the bassinet without Mom being present. She dropped the baby on the floor in her attempt to pick him up.

These are just a few examples of infant susceptibility to falls. There are certainly many more, but I believe the incidents I have cited illustrate the extreme danger falls pose for very small children, as well as the value of taking precautions and of keeping a watchful eye.

There are other unspecified types of accidents for which the precipitating factors are not reported. According to the NCHS (1990), 547 infants under the age of one died from unspecified accidental causes. There is also a very small number of infant deaths caused by accidents involving a hot substance or object, caustic or corrosive material, steam, and accidental poisoning from drugs or medications. In addition, there are deaths that accidentally occur during medical treatment or from abnormal reactions to substances given to a child.

CONCLUSION

The statistics show that over 950 infants under the age of one were killed in 1987 as a result of vehicular and nonvehicular accidents (NCHS, 1990). The problem of these accidental deaths becomes greater after the first twenty-eight days of life, during the postneonatal period. As we discussed earlier, accidents/accidental deaths rank very low (fourteenth) as a cause of infant mortality for the early days of life. From twenty-eight days to one year of age, accidents burst forth as the third most frequent cause of infant death.

ACCIDENTAL DEATH IN CHILDREN (AGED ONE TO FOURTEEN)

Although the death rate for children improves after the first year of life, it is still estimated that 31 percent of deaths in children aged one to four-teen are from causes related to accidents (State of the Child in New York State, 1988). Deaths from nonvehicular accidents occur as a result of fires, drownings, and falls. Deaths from vehicular accidents involve the child as a passenger in or on some type of car, truck, motorcycle, bicycle, or as a pedestrian. This is the primary cause of death for those one to fourteen years of age. In summary, of all accidents involving children aged one to fourteen, death resulting from riding as a passenger in a car that is subsequently involved in a collision constitutes the most frequent cause of childhood fatalities.

Although children in this age range are more likely to die as passengers in motor vehicles, many are fatally injured each year as pedestrians and as cyclists (pedal cyclists). Children aged five to nine seem especially prone to injuries as pedestrians; in this age group more deaths resulted from pedestrian injuries than from any other cause of injury (MMWR, July 6, 1990). Youngsters ten to fourteen are killed more frequently on bicycles than are younger children. It is also noted that ten- to fourteen-year-olds have more fatalities on motorcycles or mini-bikes than children one to nine years of age. The death rate for male children tends to be higher than for females with regard to all accidents in this age group involving motor vehicles (NCHS, 1990). The sale of three-wheel all-terrain vehicles (ATVs) was banned in 1988 because they were deemed unsafe. However, four-wheel ATV's were not affected. One study reports that these four-wheel vehicles are perhaps just as dangerous. The researchers examining injuries associated with ATVs conclude that children younger than sixteen should not be allowed to operate them because these adolescents are not developmentally capable of driving the ATVs safely (Dolon et al., 1989). States with the densest populations tend to have the highest mortality rates for motor vehicle accidents in children from this age group. There is some variation as to the cause and frequency of accidental deaths; however, accidents are across the board the leading cause of death among these children, and accidents involving motor vehicles are the most frequent cause of death.

The second leading cause of accidental death in the one-to-fourteen-year age group is not as straightforward as motor vehicle accidents, which are prevalent at all age levels. For nonvehicular accidents only, I divide the group into one- to four-year-olds and five- to fourteen-year-olds (see tables 1 and 2 in chapter 1). In one- to four-year-olds, the second leading cause of accidental death is fires. Between seven and eight hundred children under the age of five and approximately five hundred children aged six to fourteen died from fires (NCHS, 1990). Thus, the death rate from fires in the one- to four-year-old group is somewhat higher than that of older children. In 1982, almost 45 percent of all persons under the age of twenty who died as a result of fires were between one and four years of age. Most of these fire-related deaths resulted from house fires (Miller et al., 1986).

Death from fire happens for a variety of reasons. In many instances children playing with matches or lighters start house fires. In addition, dwellings that don't have working smoke detectors or fire alarms can effectively prevent nearby adults from rescuing a child before the fire burns out of control. These detectors save lives, but even in locations where regulations require smoke detectors to be in place, they are not always maintained. What needless tragedy!

I remember the time that my small brother and sister were playing "church" one day. They found a candle, lit it, and then held their church service under the bed in one of their rooms. The candle ignited the blanket and bedspread. Frightened by what they had done, they hid in the closet. My grandmother, who was downstairs washing breakfast dishes, thought they were just playing quietly. She was horrified when she suddenly smelled smoke. Fortunately, she got the children out of the room, called the fire department, and attempted to put out the fire. This is just one example of how carefully we must watch children in the one- to four-year-old age group. For many of these youngsters, matches and lighters are irresistible "toys."

Drowning causes about six hundred to seven hundred deaths in children one to four years of age and results in almost six hundred deaths in the five-to-fourteen age group. Male children are more likely to die from both causes than are female children. African-American children seem more at risk of death by fire, whereas white children have a greater risk from drowning.

Death by drowning often occurs because small children wander into a nearby pool at a time in their lives when they cannot swim. However, these children could just as easily drown in a bathtub if left unattended. My own son, when he was three, went to a nearby public pool with his aunt. He jumped off the side into the deepest end and was completely submerged. My sister, usually alert, didn't notice immediately. However, in a few seconds she realized he was in the water and that he was drowning. I, of course, am thankful she reacted quickly to that emergency. It saved his life. I was foolish to let my son go near a pool without a life preserver, and immediately after this life-threatening episode, I enrolled him in swimming lessons.

Airway obstruction from foreign objects claimed 118 children under the age of five years in 1987. It is the fourth most prevalent cause of death in that age. Inviting objects that can be popped into a small child's mouth may block a windpipe quite easily. If the object cannot be dislodged, it ultimately causes the child to suffocate. Food, small objects, or toys can be responsible. For instance, if a child is given food that he or she is unable to chew properly or is too large to swallow, it can become an obstruction.

The fourth most prevalent type of tragedy in five- to fourteen-year-old children is the accidental discharge of a firearm, which careless adults often leave loaded and within easy reach. The incidence of childhood death caused by younger children playing with firearms and accidentally killing themselves or a playmate is increasing at an alarming rate. As a result, some states are trying to initiate stiff penalties for adults who leave loaded guns within a child's easy grasp. In 1987, thirty-six children under the age of five died as a result of handguns and unspecified firearms (NCHS, 1990). When we examine gun-related deaths for children aged five to fourteen, the numbers are even more disturbing. In 1987, over two hundred children in this older age group perished as a result of an accident involving a firearm.

Falls are the fifth leading cause of accidental death in children in the one- to fourteen-year-old age group.

Accidental poisonings stand as the sixth most frequent form of death in this age range. It is apparent that the most frequently occurring poisonings are from ingesting medications and solvents (or other household cleaners) and inhaling the vapors from such solvents as well as natural gas or other gaseous substances such as carbon monoxide (NCHS, 1990). These poisonings seem to occur more often in and around the child's home. Fatal poisonings associated with medicines primarily involve analgesics (pain medications) and antipyretics (i.e., aspirin or medications for fever). In a portion of these accidental drug poisonings, the specific medication or chemical compound causing the death is not stated. Although childhood mortality due to poisoning has decreased in recent years, morbidity associated with poisoning in this age group remains a major health problem. In 1987, the American Association of Poison Control Center's national data collection system received reports of 731,954 poisoning exposures. Twenty-two of these children died and 107,844 others became ill (MMWR, March 17, 1989). When I was a child, my next door neighbor's five-year-old son died from taking his father's pain medication. He ate all the pills in the bottle, went to sleep, and never woke up. His parents found him dead with the empty bottle laying in the corner of his bedroom.

One all-too-frequent form of accidental death for those aged one to fourteen is electrocution. Over fifty children died in 1987 as a result of electrical accidents of one sort or another (NCHS, 1990). Uncovered electrical outlets, exposed wiring, and household appliances can prove lethal to the curious, playful, or imaginative child. Another way a child can be seriously hurt or even killed is from using electrical appliances in an unsafe manner. When my daughter was younger, she thought she could bring her hairdryer to the tub and dry her hair while she bathed. Fortunately, I intercepted her and explained that she could seriously injure or even kill herself if she attempted to follow her initial plan.

CONCLUSION

As children grow, their environment extends beyond the home, making it far more difficult to control the safety of their surroundings. However, the vast majority of accidents can be prevented if adults look for, point out, and then correct structural safety hazards in and around home, school, and play areas. It is important that children become aware of and learn to recognize dangers in their environment. We all want our kids to feel comfortable exploring their surroundings—how else are they to learn about their world than by experiencing it firsthand?—but we also need to ensure to the best of our ability their physical safety.

At greatest risk for accidental injury in the one-to-fourteen age group are children from low-income and poorly educated families who live in inadequate or substandard housing where risks lurk in every room, and those children who live in unusually stressful home environments where they are distracted from their own personal safety. If we control for all variables except gender, a fascinating fact emerges: Statistics indicate that male children run a greater risk of accidental death than do females in this age group. However, accidents are responsible for about 12 percent of all childhood deaths (Miller et al., 1986).

ACCIDENTAL DEATH IN TEENAGERS (AGED FIFTEEN TO NINETEEN)

The late teen years are a time when many young lives are lost. As a result of accidents of all types, approximately 8,528 teens aged fifteen to nineteen lost their lives in 1987. Total injuries from accidental shootings of all types and from drownings are very high during the teen years primarily because teenagers often take risks that older, more mature people would not. As with younger children, if the home environment is very stressful or they live in inadequate or substandard housing, the risk of accidental death among teenagers increased dramatically. In addition, the use and abuse of alcohol and drugs by teenagers increase their risk of accident fatalities (Miller et al., 1986). Again gender plays a part in this age group: male teenagers seem to be more at risk than females for all types of accidental death (NCHS, 1990).

Motor Vehicle Accidents

The number one cause of accidental death among teenagers is automobile mishaps, with white males being particularly at risk. Two out of every five deaths in older adolescents are related to car accidents, and in the majority of these the driver tests positive for alcohol abuse (Miller et al., 1986). Driving while intoxicated represents a major threat to our teenage children.

According to the latest available statistics, 6,805 teenagers between the ages of fifteen and nineteen died as a result of motor vehicle accidents of all types in 1987 (NCHS, 1990). This includes drivers and passengers as well as pedestrians and cyclists involved in accidents with motor vehicles. Of these fatalities, 4,798 were male and 2,007 were female. As in years past, the death toll for white teenagers in this age group is extremely high, representing 6,134 (or more than 90 percent) of the total motor vehicle fatalities. This can be compared to 495 fatalities (or slightly more than 7 percent) among African-Americans and 176 deaths among teens of other races and/or ethnic groups. Of these fatalities, 2,337 were drivers of a motor vehicle, 1,845 were passengers, 467 were motorcycle drivers, and 100 were passengers on a motorcycle. The largest number of fatalities involving motorcycles is for white males and females in this age group. The remaining fatalities involved teens whose role in the accident was not specified by the National Center for Health Statistics (1990).

While the number of teenage lives lost in motor vehicle accidents is unacceptably high, there are many other dangers facing our youngsters in their teen years. Many lives are lost as a result of traffic accidents involving teens on bicycles: in the fifteen-to-nineteen age group, 156 teens died in such accidents during 1987. There were also 433 teen pedestrians who were hit by some type of motor vehicle and subsequently died as a result of the injuries they sustained.

It should come as no surprise that for accidents involving motor vehicles, those states with the densest populations tend to have the highest death rates (NCHS, 1990).

Additionally, eighty-seven teens died from water transport accidents involving boats or related marine vehicles. Again, a disproportionately large number of the victims, sixty-eight in all or 78 percent, were white males.

When I was a teenager, five young men sixteen to eighteen years of age were killed in an automobile accident. They had been drinking heavily at a tavern and left very intoxicated. At the time, the legal drinking age was eighteen, but they had faked their identification to ensure being served. The driver, whom I'll name Joe, was sixteen and the youngest of the five. I remember him as one of the funniest, most sociable guys in my town. Joe and his friends were challenged by some other teens in the tavern; they agreed to race along a very winding stretch of country road to determine who had the fastest car. When they raced down the road, the challengers' car slowed down enough to maintain control. But Joe, too drunk to steer clear of hazards, never made one of the turns. He sped into a heavily wooded area at over a hundred miles per hour and hit a tree. The car was demolished and Joe was killed instantly, as were three of his passengers. One young man did survive the crash. That carnage happened over twenty years ago, but despite the horror and pain such tragedies cause families and friends each year in this country, these incidents have not served to deter our young people from mixing drinking and driving.

Other Accidents

The second leading cause of accidental death in teens is drowning. Over four hundred teen victims were reported in 1987 (NCHS, 1990), and more than 90 percent of these drownings involved males in this fifteen- to nineteen-year-old age group.

The third most prevalent category of accidental teenage death involved handguns or other firearms. Over two hundred teens lost their lives in such incidents.

Poisonings of various kinds constitute the fourth most common cause of accidental death during the teen years: they accounted for 425 fatalities in 1987. These poisonings occurred as a result of ingesting solid or liquid substances, drugs or medications, and the inhalation of lethal gases or vapors. The majority of deaths attributed to accidental poisoning from drugs can be divided into three subcategories: those related to illicit drugs, those due to the misuse of over-the-counter medications, and those related to prescription medications. The taking of drugs in one of these three forms accounted for 304 (71.5 percent) of the 425 deaths attributed to accidental poisoning. The National Center for Health Statistics examines these accidental poisonings and issues information about the types of medications and drugs that are responsible for the deaths. However, they do not focus on fifteen- to nineteen-year-olds. Their figures report on young people aged fifteen to twenty-four. Therefore, the information provided by the NCHS covers a larger number of deaths than we have been addressing. However, this information is important and I feel that it does have direct implications for our fifteen-to-nineteen age group since they represent about 30 percent of the deaths within this category. These data can provide some insights into the kinds of drugs most often responsible for accidental poisonings that are medication related.

In 1986, the leading causes of fatal unintentional drug poisonings were opiates and related narcotics, and local anesthetics including cocaine. Most of the fatal poisonings by other solids and liquids in this age group were due to alcohol ingestion. Exposure to motor vehicle exhaust accounted for nearly half the deaths due to unintentional poisoning by gas and vapors (MMWR, March 17, 1990).

The major type of legal drug involved in accidental deaths occurring in this group consists of analgesics, antipyretics, and drugs of a similar nature (NCHS, 1990). Drugs that act to depress the central nervous system were found in the bodies of the largest group of victims aged fifteen to twenty-four.

As with other age groups, fire-related deaths ranked fifth among the leading causes of death in this group of young people. Falls ranked sixth in terms of teen death. Ninety-three children in this age group fell to their death. The majority were from falls between two levels (NCHS, 1990).

Additionally, there were various unclassified accidents and those for which the principle cause was not determined; these, too, cause a significant proportion of deaths in our teen children.

CONCLUSION

In summary, over eight thousand fifteen- to nineteen-year-olds die each year from accidents of all types. The death rate for these young people is roughly eighty-five per one hundred thousand in the population. These figures, alarming in their own right, become even more distressing when it is learned that the death rate for males is double that for females. The overall death rate from accidents in general for African-American males is higher than for any other group in this age range, although white males are the most frequent victims of motor vehicle accident fatalities. A total of 15,615 fifteen- to nineteen-year-olds died in 1987 from all causes. As we can see, accidents are responsible for over one-half the teen deaths in this age group. In chapter 4 we will look at other causes that claim the lives of our teenagers, but none draws our attention more than the senseless and unnecessary deaths attributed to accidents.

4

Fatal Illness

INTRODUCTION

Illness, disease, and various medical conditions take the lives of many of our nation's children. Although the epidemics of the late nineteenth and early twentieth centuries have been controlled and for the most part eradicated due to advances in medical care, there are still diseases and physical conditions that rank high among the causes of childhood death. Although these diseases and physical conditions afflict all age groups, they exact an especially heavy toll on the infant population. We will look at these conditions for all age groups but especially in this younger, more susceptible population.

When discussing illnesses, we will touch upon only the most common varieties. Each age group will be considered because the diseases and conditions vary from group to group and their rank in terms of impact on the death toll is different for each age level.

INFANTS

We know from our previous discussion that infants under the age of one are classified in two ways: for the first twenty-eight days of life they are considered neonates, while the period from twenty-eight days to the end of the eleventh month (or one year of age) is classified as the postneonatal period. This distinction is important because the primary causes of death are different in each period. In the neonatal period, congenital anomalies, or birth defects, are the most prevalent cause of death, followed by disorders related to low birth weight. In the postneonatal periods, Sudden Infant Death Syndrome (SIDS) is the leading cause of death from disease, followed by congenital anomalies and defects. When the two periods are considered together, congenital anomalies, SIDS, disorders related to low birth weight, and acute respiratory distress syndrome are the leading causes of death from disease under the age of one. They also happen to be the leading causes of death *in general* for this age group (NCHS, 1990).

Let's look at each of these causes in greater detail.

Congenital Anomalies

In 1987, 7,884 infants died from congenital anomalies in their first year of life, which means that for 1987 the United States posted an infant mortality rate of 207 per 100,000 live births (NCHS, 1990). The most lethal type of congenital anomalies are those associated with the structure of the heart, which claimed more than 2,000 infants in their first eleven months of life (NCHS, 1990). Over one-quarter of all infant deaths from birth defects involve some malformation of this organ.

During pregnancy the baby's vital organs develop to the point that the child can be independent of the womb. While in utero, however, the baby's developing heart is especially vulnerable to conditions that affect its mother's health. Birth defects of the heart interfere with the flow of oxygen to vital tissues, and without oxygen to the tissues and vital organs, the baby will die. The most frequently occurring heart defect is *patent ductus arteriosus,* a condition involving an open blood vessel located between the major artery (pulmonary) that brings the infant's blood back to the heart and the artery (aorta) that takes fresh blood (containing oxygen) from the heart to the vital organs. In *patent ductus arteriosus,* the small connecting vessel between the aorta and the pulmonary artery does not close at birth thus allowing the blood from both arteries to mix. Ultimately not enough blood gets reoxygenated to meet the body's demand. This is the most prevalent form of heart defect, and it occurs more frequently in females (Whaley and Wong, 1987).

Other heart defects involve openings between the chambers or sections of the heart such as atrial septal defect (top chambers of heart) or ventricular septal defect (bottom chambers of heart). Again, they interfere with the heart pumping enough oxygen-rich blood to the vital organs. In addition, there are heart defects in which arteries and veins that feed and drain the heart narrow significantly so that the blood flow through this structure is diminished. Sometimes the valves regulating the flow of blood through the heart's compartments are too narrow, fail to close and open properly, or do not develop at all during pregnancy. If any one of these conditions arises, blood cannot flow through the heart in a normal manner. Because of its crucial role in the transport of oxygenated blood to vital body organs and tissues, the proper functioning of the heart is essential to an infant's survival. The defects mentioned above are the most common dangers to children in the first few days of life and they are very often lethal (NCHS, 1990).

If the link to heredity or genetic origins (Servonsky and Opas, 1987) is set aside, the reason heart defects occur is often because the mother's health has been poor during pregnancy. An illness contracted while she is pregnant may disturb the fetus's development. Viruses such as rubella (German Measles) or herpes can affect how the unborn baby's heart develops. Other causes of these heart defects are related to the side-effects of drugs. For precisely this reason pregnant women should consult a pediatrician before taking any drug or medication.

The second most common type of congenital anomaly that results in infant death consists of defects in the childs respiratory system or breathing apparatus. If the specific defect or malformation is serious enough, it may be life threatening. The death rate for respiratory defects is twenty-nine per one hundred thousand live births. Over one thousand infants die in their first year from these defects (NCHS, 1990). Again, illness or other conditions that affect the mother's health during pregnancy can cause these birth defects in her unborn child. Regrettably, there are many more types of congenital defects, all of which can cause infant death, but we've touched on the most serious and the most frequently occurring ones.

Sudden Infant Death Syndrome (SIDS)

Often termed "crib death," Sudden Infant Death Syndrome is the second leading cause of death in infants under the age of one. It is an illness the cause of which is still not clear. According to the National SIDS Foundation (1987), the syndrome can be defined as "the sudden and unexpected death of an apparently healthy infant for whom a thorough post-mortem investigation including an autopsy fails to demonstrate an adequate cause of death." Though theories abound regarding the actual causes of these unexpected deaths, there are several risk factors to keep in mind:

1. prematurity, low birth weight, and being one infant in a multiple birth;
2. periods of apnea or no respiration, which require treatment or medical intervention;
3. respiratory distress syndrome;
4. a history of SIDS in the family.

The cause of SIDS remains a mystery. What we do know is that most deaths occur while the child is asleep (Servonsky and Opas, 1987). Prior to their death, some infants did have an upper respiratory tract infection, but at the time of autopsy these did not appear severe enough to have resulted in an obstruction of the airway sufficient to cause death. Total airway closure seems to be the cause of death; however, what actually produces that closure cannot be isolated to highlight any one single cause.

Current theories regarding SIDS attempt to trace its cause to a virus, airway narrowing, pneumonia, and immune deficiencies, to name a few (Servonsky and Opas, 1987). Adults and parents can probably help most by being aware and informed about this type of problem and by providing financial and/or political support for further research on this and other such diseases/syndromes. Some research indicates that siblings of SIDS victims have a 2 percent increased risk of infant death from this disease. Careful counseling may be suggested for parents who have already experienced the pain of a SIDS-related death (Guntheroth et al., 1990).

Low-Birth-Weight Infants

Low birth weight is an underlying condition the complications of which claim the third largest number of infants overall, and it ranks third among causes of death related to a disease or medical condition. High-risk infants are most often classified according to size or weight, by what point in the pregnancy they are born, and by the type of health problems they have at birth. The more common health problems associated with low birth weight seem closely related to the immaturity of organs and body systems, which are unable to function once the fetus has left the womb. Formerly, weight at birth was thought to be a good indicator of maturity. Therefore, if a baby was five pounds at birth, it was considered full-term. However, data have shown that the rate at which an infant grows in the womb is not the same for all women because other factors such as maternal disease or health practices can affect growth within the uterus. To summarize, low-birth-weight infants have more problems and are at a greater risk of death because either the baby was born too soon or the mother's condition/status prevented normal growth within the womb. In either case, the baby is at risk and has a poorer chance of survival (Whaley and Wong, 1987).

Respiratory Distress Syndrome

The fourth type of medical problem that results in infant death is acute respiratory distress syndrome (RDS), so named because it applies to respiratory dysfunction in very young infants and is related to lung maturation (Whaley and Wong, 1987). It also ranks fourth among all causes of death in infants. Usually seen in pre-term or premature infants, RDS was responsible for 3,283 infant deaths in 1987; and even if treated, it carries the greatest risk of long-term neurological complications.

Infections

Newborns are highly susceptible to infections (Whaley and Wong, 1987), the seventh largest cause of death in babies under one year of age (NCHS, 1990). When infants leave the hospital they are very vulnerable to many types of infection and require prompt medical attention when they are ill. Without adequate care, we lose many to these diseases, which are treatable if medical attention is sought early (Druschel and Hale, 1987). A virus that causes a significant number of deaths (2,736) in infants under one year of age is Respiratory Syncytial Virus, a major cause of lower respiratory infections and respiratory deaths in infants. Since the health burden of this type of infection is escalating, there should be some impetus to develop a vaccine and vaccination program. (Anderson et al., 1990).

Septicemia

Septicemia is a potentially lethal condition ranking thirteenth among the leading causes of death in infants (NCHS, 1990). It generally occurs as the result of a bacteria from an infected site in the body that invades the blood stream causing a serious infection.

Meningitis

This infection of the membrane covering the brain or spinal cord ranks fifteenth among the deadliest illnesses to which infants are susceptible (NCHS, 1990). Meningitis is caused by a variety of bacteria that gain access to the brain tissue usually during the course of a respiratory infection. The bacteria multiply and cause serious inflammation. The obvious potential consequence of meningitis is death; however, other problems (such as permanent brain and nerve damage) can also occur.

SUMMARY

Infants under the age of one year are susceptible to a great many medical conditions, health problems, or diseases, some of which are the major causes of death in this age group. As we discussed, many of the conditions that kill infants are contingent on maternal health practices or the care the mother receives during pregnancy. The top four causes of infant death overlap because congenital anomalies (birth defects) are related to the mother's health. Low-birth-weight babies seem to have a higher incidence of congenital anomalies and acute respiratory distress syndrome. The condition known as SIDS may be related to any of these health risks, but the causes are still not clear. We do know that disease and the infant's medical condition are clearly the primary factors associated with the deaths of youngsters less than one year of age. As we have shown, these are strongly linked to maternal health and lifestyle.

MEDICAL CONDITIONS AND ILLNESS IN CHILDREN (AGED ONE TO FOURTEEN)

Cancer and congenital anomalies rank high among the leading causes of death for children aged one to fourteen. Some common forms of cancer in children, with which the reader may be familiar, are leukemia, lymphomas (tumors of the lymph nodes), and osteosarcoma (bone cancer). Despite the advances in medical technology, congenital birth defects still account for a substantial number of deaths in this age range. These two serious health problems rank second (cancer) and third (congenital anomalies) among the leading causes of death in this group of children (State of the Child in New York State, 1988).

Cancer

According to the latest statistics (NCHS, 1990), cancer in all its forms claimed over two thousand victims between the ages of one and fourteen in 1987. Cancers of the lymphatic and hematopoietic systems are the second most prevalent forms of childhood cancer resulting in death for children in this age range. Lymphatic tumors are cell growths involving lymph vessels and nodes. The lymphatic system is an accessory to the blood vascular system. The hematopoietic system is responsible for the formation of the components in blood. Of all forms of cancers affecting our young people, leukemia is the most common variety, occurring more frequently in white children than in African-American youngsters and in males more often than in females (Whaley and Wong, 1987). The different types of leukemia are classified according to the types of blood cells that microscopic examination indicates are being affected: different leukemias attack different types of cells. As a disease that destroys blood cells, leukemia results in anemia, infection, and/or bleeding because these cells nourish body tissues, protect the body against infection, and/or help the blood to clot normally so that abnormal bleeding does not occur.

In recent years, leukemia has become one of the general forms of cancer that has experienced dramatic improvements in survival rates (Poplock, 1985). Forty years ago a child diagnosed with leukemia might well have died in two or three months. Today, with all our advanced treatments, medical science has effected very dramatic cure rates. For some forms of leukemia major research centers have achieved a 60 percent rate of survival after five years. Although the majority of children with this disease may be cured (Poplack, 1985), leukemia still remains a leading cause of death among the young.

Malignant tumors of other organs and various body parts, together with brain tumors, rank collectively as the third most frequently occurring types of cancerous growths in children.

Osteosarcoma is the most frequently encountered type of bone cancer in children aged one to fourteen years (Whaley and Wong, 1987). The most common initial site of origin for this cancer is in the long bones of the leg. However, bones in the arm, pelvis, and other extremities can be primary sites for the disease to begin. Again, the long-term survival of these children has improved dramatically. Some reports show a 50 percent long-term survival rate (Whaley and Wong, 1987). Nonetheless, many children do not survive. Therefore, osteosarcoma contributes to the number of children who die as a result of cancer.

Cancer is the leading cause of death from disease in children one to fourteen years of age, and the second leading cause of death in general in this age group. (Accidents, as noted above, are the leading cause of death in this age group.) The mortality rates from childhood cancer have declined, but we still lose many children to the ravages of this disease.

A dear friend's seven-year-old son was diagnosed with a type of leukemia. The child was treated at a comprehensive cancer center and now, after several years, he is still in remission. This young man is truly heroic, for his cure involved many visits to the hospital, all of which he endured with courage. He is a success story. Unfortunately, such success is not achieved for all types of cancer.

The cause(s) of cancer(s) is not yet known, but some risk factors have been identified. For instance, certain drugs when given to pregnant women caused cancer in their children. Diethystilbesterol is probably the best known of these. It had been widely prescribed to prevent miscarriage. Later, it was discovered that the drug caused cancer of the vagina in many of the female offspring. Other risk factors for cancer in the general population, such as smoking and overexposure to sunlight, radiation, and certain chemicals (e.g., dioxin), have been widely publicized over the past ten to twenty years (Whaley and Wong, 1987). Knowledge of these risk factors as well as others may help in our search for a cure; in the meantime, understanding the risks can help us avoid the circumstances with which cancer is strongly linked.

Congenital Anomalies

The defects that occur during the development of the fetus in the womb cause many deaths in infants at birth and in their first year of life. However, this death toll remains high throughout the childhood years. Congenital anomalies involving the heart and the circulatory system remain the most lethal type of defect in this age group. Such congenital conditions were responsible for over nine hundred deaths among youngsters one to fourteen years of age. These conditions may be detected at birth, may occur as a result of another chronic disease, and/or cause steady deterioration in a child's physical health, which ultimately leads to death. On the other hand, they may also remain undetected at birth and cause death years later, at a time when the child is much older. Congenital defects may be hereditary (i.e., genetic) or the result of some disturbance during the baby's development in the womb, possibly caused by the mother's health habits or physical condition during pregnancy.

Other Diseases

Diseases or conditions of the nervous system, heart and circulatory system, and the respiratory tract rank third, fourth, and fifth, respectively, in terms of childhood illnesses that result in fatalities, and fourth, fifth, and sixth when overall causes of death in this age group are considered.

The most common diseases are those involving the nervous system. *Meningitis* is the most prevalent form of nervous-system disorder in infants, as we have already discussed. Other nerve disorders that may contribute to the death of a child are cerebral palsy and epilepsy (NCHS, 1990). *Cerebral palsy* is a conditon that results from an injury to the baby's brain during pregnancy, delivery, or as the result of a severe head trauma. The cause cannot always be clearly defined but it is characterized by spastic-type movements. Sometimes it remains unnoticed early in a child's life but becomes more apparant when the youngster does not demonstrate normal physical developmental movements appropriate to its age. For instance, the child may not be able to sit up, gain head control, or grasp objects. The parents or physician may notice spastic, uncontrollable movements in the child's extremities or a tightness of the leg muscles. There is no specific cure for cerebral palsy, which is the most frequent cause of childhood physical disability. These children need physical, medical, and speech therapy to reach their optimum potential. Very often they contract lethal respiratory diseases because of limited activity and increased susceptibility to infectious processes.

Epilepsy is a brain disorder in which nerve cells misfire and cause a variety of seizure characteristics. The disease can be caused by a number of factors such as head injury, lead toxicity, or infections. All types of seizures can be controlled by drug therapy, but they can be fatal if complications arise. For example, an individual who is having a seizure can suffocate on his vomit. If the person experiences a type of seizure that renders him unconscious, a fall or spastic movement could result in severe injury.

Once, while I was parking my car at the university, I noticed a young girl, probably in her teens, standing by the curb. She looked distracted, but since I was on my way to class, I didn't take full notice of her situation. As soon as I got out of the car, she collapsed to the ground from a standing position, became unconscious, and began having a seizure with jerking, uncontrolled movements of her extremities. I tried to cradle her head and protect her from injury while a friend who had been riding with me ran for help. When the emergency crew arrived, the young girl's seizure had subsided and she went off with them. I have often wondered what happened to her because her head hit the sidewalk so hard as she fell to the ground; it seemed likely that she had suffered some type of head injury. This situation illustrates how a child might die of injuries sustained during an epileptic seizure.

One nerve disease that is very common in school-age children is *Reye's*

Syndrome. It is an acute and often fatal disease that infects the tissues of the brain and causes severe swelling and other life-threatening symptoms. It is thought to occur in children who are recovering from a viral infection. The exact cause is not known but some studies indicate that it seems to occur more frequently in children who receive aspirin during a bout of flu. Therefore, physicians usually recommend that aspirin not be given to children except under proper medical supervision.

In conclusion, the NCHS (1990) indicates that over one thousand children died in 1987 as a result of diseases related to the nervous system. Meningitis is the most prevalent cause with various other degenerative diseases a close second. This brief discussion certainly does not cover all conditions of the nervous-system, only the most pervasive and life-threatening.

The next most prevalent type of lethal disease or disorder in children is associated with the heart and circulatory system. Some of these conditions result from bacteria that invade various tissues of the heart thereby causing infection. One that many people are familiar with is *rheumatic fever*. It usually involves a specific type of streptococcal (bacteria or germ) infection that seems to trigger the symptoms of the disease, which involves an inflammation of various parts of the heart. However, the exact cause is unclear. For some children there is a hereditary disposition toward this disease, the incidence of which appears to have increased during the past half century. Children five to fifteen seem to be at most risk for the disease, and it is more common in girls and in African-Americans. Other forms of heart disease are endocarditis, pericarditis, and myocarditis, which are inflammations of the various layers of heart tissue.

There are other diseases with cardiac complications or side effects that may eventually result in death. Some of the more well-known of these diseases result from chromosomal abnormalities like Down's syndrome or are hereditary like cystic fibrosis or sickle cell anemia. These diseases may predispose their young victims to severe cardiac problems and even death.

In conclusion, over eight hundred children between the ages of one and fourteen died as a result of cardiac problems in 1987 (NCHS, 1990).

The last type of disease process we will review is that involving the respiratory system. By far, *pneumonia* is the most prevalent and potentially lethal illness of the respiratory system. Over seven hundred children died from pneumonia in 1987 (NCHS, 1990). Pneumonia is an acute inflammation of the lungs caused by a wide array of bacteria and viruses. Very simply, the lungs become congested, which severely impairs their ability to breathe thus reducing the level of oxygen to the body. If the infection is severe enough, it can kill a child.

SUMMARY: CHILDHOOD ILLNESS

Although cancers and congenital defects rank second and third respectively among the leading causes of death in children aged one to fourteen, the preceding section has shown that there are many other serious and often fatal conditions that place our children at risk. Bacterial and viral infections can also cause death among these youngsters but their mortality rates are significantly lower, though they do exceed the death rate for homicide in this age group. (It ranks seventh.) One infectious disease that is affecting infants and children at an alarming rate is, of course, AIDS. It is not as yet a major cause of death in children, though the rate at which AIDS among youngsters is growing deserves special attention. Therefore, it will be addressed separately when additional threats to the health and safety of our young people are considered in an upcoming section of this chapter. At the beginning of this century, there were other childhood diseases that exacted a terrible toll in terms of young lives. Many of these diseases have been practically eradicated owing to the development of vaccines, and public health programs throughout the United States have provided these vaccines to children over the years. For a time, the extraordinary expense involved in producing and distributing the needed serum threatened the effectiveness of these immunization programs. However, more federal aid to programs is being provided (Hamilton and Garland, 1988) and we can only hope that all children will have access to these immunizations.

All children must be immunized before entering school. However, the diseases that the vaccines are supposed to prevent in school-age children, if caught by an infant, could prove fatal. Therefore, delaying a baby's shots until the child goes to school could have fatal consequences for an infant who has contact with children experiencing active cases of such diseases as mumps or whooping cough. Most public health officials believe infants should complete their initial immunizations by the time they are two years of age. There is evidence that the number of children receiving immunizations is decreasing rather than increasing. If this trend continues, we will have outbreaks of disease in this country the likes of which we have not seen for several decades.

Therefore, although instances of communicable diseases such as dyptheria and polio has been practically eradicated, we should not forget the lessons of the past.

DISEASE IN ADOLESCENTS
(FIFTEEN TO NINETEEN YEARS OF AGE)

Youths in this group are largely past the age at which death from congenital defects and life-threatening illnesses of infancy place them in serious jeopardy (State of the Child in New York State, 1988). In fact, the number of deaths due to congenital anomalies in this age group is less than 300 (NCHS, 1990). However, cancer still causes about 810 deaths during the middle to late teens (NCHS, 1990). These young people have not yet reached adulthood and do not suffer from the degenerative diseases associated with more physically mature individuals. Yet, many of the bad habits typical of adult behavior, such as substance abuse, poor nutrition, and smoking, can set the stage for illness and death in later life. Comparatively speaking, the death rate of every illness contracted or diagnosed during these adolescent years is totally eclipsed by the fatalities resulting from accidents, suicide, and homicide, the three most frequent causes of death in this age group. However, according to the latest reports, the sexual practices of teens may render them more at risk for AIDS than otherwise thought (WNY AIDS Newsletter, 1990). It is increasing in prevalence for all age groups, and by the time this book goes to press, it may be a leading cause of death in children in this age group because of their proclivity for increased sexual activity and their disregard of "safe" (use of condoms) sexual practices.

GROWING THREATS

AIDS

Having looked at the most current and devastating illnesses that afflict children, we will now turn to potential threats that may further hurt our children's chances of survival if they remain unchallenged.

In 1981, Acquired Immune Deficiency Syndrome was isolated and identified, and since that time the number of cases has steadily increased. In New York City alone, the number of cases has increased 655 percent from 22 in 1983 to 166 in 1986 (State of the Child in New York State, 1988). This disease is contagious in that it can be spread by blood-to-blood or semen-to-blood contact. Sexual contact with an infected person and sharing intravenous drug paraphernalia are the leading modes of transmission among adults. Small children contract AIDS primarily from their infected mothers before or during birth. A small number have contracted it through blood transfusions prior to the present nationwide screening of blood products.

As of June 1987, a total of fifty-one children from birth through age thirteen had been diagnosed with AIDS. The incidence of AIDS among African-American infants in New York City is 54 percent; Hispanic, 25 percent; and 20 percent for white infants (State of Child in New York State, 1988). Approximately thirty adolescents have been diagnosed in New York City; that number may increase dramatically due to increases in drug use and sexual activity among these children (State of Child in New York State, 1988).

None of the above figures includes the unknown numbers of children with AIDS-Related Complex (ARC), which is a less severe form of AIDS. Although children with the disease have symptoms similar to those seen in AIDS victims, they do not contract the other types of infections (e.g., pneumonias) that AIDS victims normally experience. It is estimated that there are three to five children with ARC for every child diagnosed with AIDS. In New York City alone, AIDS became the fifth leading cause of death in children age one to four (State of the Child in New York State, 1988). This is why AIDS and its related illnesses deserve our attention now even though on the national level these conditions do not pose as major a threat to our children as other causes of death currently under study. However, the growth rate of AIDS is unparalleled and the statistics are frightening for that very reason.

In reviewing the latest statistics available to the National Center for Health Statistics (1990), the states with the greatest number of deaths among children that could be directly attributed to AIDS are ranked in the following order: New York (first), California (second), and New Jersey (third). Nationwide, forty-one children under the age of one year died from AIDS in 1987. Over five hundred children aged one to twenty-four died from this disease in that same year. Over half of these deaths were in the African-American population (NCHS, 1990).

In 1988, state and local health departments reported 583 cases of children diagnosed as having AIDS. During this period, African-Americans and Hispanics continued to have the highest incidence. As of December 31, 1988, 1,346 reported AIDS patients were less than thirteen years of age. Over one-half were males, and 82 percent were younger than five years of age when diagnosed. Seventy-eight percent acquired the disease from their mothers, 13 percent contracted AIDS from blood transfusions, and about 6 percent became infected from blood products. The remaining cases were those in which the causes could not be determined. Over half of the mothers

(54 percent) who infected their children were intravenous drug users, 19 percent had had sexual relations with an IV drug user, 7 percent had had sex with a man infected with the AIDS virus, and 2 percent had contracted AIDS from blood transfusions. Again, some of the modes of transmission for the disease in selected individuals could not be identified (MMWR, June 23, 1989). In conclusion, 55 percent of all children diagnosed with AIDS have since died. Eighty-five percent of all persons diagnosed with AIDS prior to 1986 have died as of 1989 (MMWR, June 23, 1989).

AIDS is climbing the charts as one of the most lethal diseases known. It demands our attention. Therefore, although not as yet a high-ranking cause of death in children, it certainly threatens to become one in the near future.

Lead Poisoning

There are other health conditions in childhood that do not rank particularly high among the causes of death but do nevertheless bear watching. For example, lead poisoning found in children who live in substandard or unsafe living conditions can result in permanent disability and even death. Poisoning as a consequence of high levels of lead—an extremely toxic substance—in the body usually occurs when small children eat paint chips that have fallen off the walls or ceiling. Illness can also occur if youngsters lick or suck their fingers after touching painted plaster in older buildings where the paint contains large quantities of lead. Newer paints (manufactured after 1960) do not have high percentages of lead in their composition. However, the victims of lead poisoning are often housed in older, dilapidated buildings where the paint still remains from many years before. Unfortunately, children often eat these paint chips or bits of plaster and subsequently develop high levels of lead in their young bodies. When the lead content in the body registers at a high level, it can cause a variety of health problems, including nerve and brain damage or even death (Miller et al., 1986). Children who live in substandard housing where the paint is old run the greatest risk of falling victim to lead poisoning. They should be screened for lead content in their bodies by their local health department.

Nutritional Deficiencies

Recent trends based on available data indicate that iron-deficiency anemia may be very prevalent in our children. This form of anemia, which is caused by insufficient dietary intake of iron, is an indicator of the health status of a population. Minority children and children from families of low socioeconomic status seem prone to this problem (Miller et al., 1986). Stunted growth—not attaining the normal physical stature for a given age—is also an indicator of society's nutritional status. As in the case of anemia, preliminary evidence indicates that this problem occurs most frequently in disadvantaged children (Miller et al., 1986). Children with chronic (long-term) anemia may be more prone to health problems and illness. Therefore, they are more at risk for early death than children without chronic anemia.

These two health problems of our disadvantaged youth indicate that a segment of our young population does not eat well enough to meet minimal standards of growth and health for their age. Inadequate nutrition makes a population more vulnerable to illness and death. The problem also poses a question regarding the health and welfare of future generations: What will be the health profile of the offspring of these nutritionally deficient youngsters as they move into their child-bearing years? A child's health status has long-term as well as short-term implications for both the child and the broader society.

It is well documented that the funding to assist programs for the disadvantaged does not reach all needy children in this country. The Hunger Prevention Act of 1988 made progress, but more needs to be done (Children's Defense Fund, 1989).

Inadequate Immunization

Many children in this country are at present inadequately immunized against disease. This lack of protection can result in outbreaks of childhood diseases, which can lead to disability and even death. It has been shown that the cost of providing immunizations ultimately saves many dollars in health care expenses (Miller et al, 1986). There is evidence to indicate that most children do not receive immunizations until they reach school age. Therefore, preschoolers who are not immunized in accordance with acceptable standards may be at risk of contracting serious illnesses.

In the case of measles, two major types of outbreaks have occurred in the United States: those among unvaccinated preschool-aged children and those among vaccinated school-aged children (MMWR, January 13, 1990). Immunization surveys conducted among the preschool populations where the outbreaks occurred demonstrated that 88 percent of the cases were among the unvaccinated children aged sixteen months to four years (MMWR,

January 13, 1990). Because of these outbreaks, the new recommendation is for a two-dose schedule given at intervals before the child is two years old (MMRW, January 13, 1990). In the case of most childhood immunizations, it is recommended that they are received before the child's second birthday (MMWR, January 13, 1990). In 1988, the Centers for Disease Control recorded 3,411 cases of measles with complications in 12 percent of the cases and three deaths (MMWR, September 1 and September 8, 1989).

In regard to mumps, the incidence has been rising since 1985, especially in older adolescents. Not all states require the mumps vaccine and, according to reports, these states have a higher incidence than those that do require the vaccine. Meningoencephalitis (infection of the membranes of the brain, spinal cord, and nervous system) and orchitis (inflammation of a testis) are potential complications of mumps (MMWR, June 9, 1989).

These outbreaks point toward the need to intensify immunization efforts and to do so at an earlier age. We must ensure that our children have the necessary protection against illness and its complications.

SUMMARY

In this chapter we have reviewed diseases and other medical conditions that claim the lives of many of our infants, children, and teens. Reviewing the medical reasons children die is both complex and disturbing. The dangers that confront our young people are considerable and indeed formidable, but research and preventive health care should go a long way toward reducing the number of young victims. Although the continuing menace of disease and other medical conditions kills far too many of our children and teens, the more significant causes of death tend to be external.

5

Suicide

FIVE- TO FOURTEEN-YEAR-OLDS

We cannot talk about the fatal risks facing our teenagers—and, yes, even our older children—without confronting the social reality of suicide. The number of young people between the ages of five and fourteen who commit suicide is a national tragedy. In 1982, over two hundred such children took their own lives and the number was projected to increase significantly by the year 2000. Recent research indicates that the rate of suicide may actually be declining (Miller et al., 1986), but, as of this date, it remains a leading cause of death in this age group (NCHS, 1990). In 1987, the latest year for which we have complete statistics, the deaths of 251 children between the ages of five and fourteen were reported as suicides. In the future, self-inflicted death may well become a major threat to the lives of children in this age group but at present it is not among the top five causes of death. In children under the age of ten, only one death could be directly attributed to suicide in 1987 (NCHS). Therefore, suicide ranks extremely low in that group. However, between the ages of ten and fourteen, it ranks about eleventh as a cause of death.

A nursing friend of mine who works with emotionally disturbed children told me that she has treated youngsters who have attempted to take their own lives even at the age of five. She was overwhelmed by how lethal their thoughts about themselves could be. It may seem hard to believe that children so young could be suicidal and make very serious attempts to end their lives. Such destructive thought processes seem beyond the comprehension of a young child. Unfortunately, they are not. A child from an unhealthy and unhappy home environment can become a suicide statistic.

FIFTEEN- TO NINETEEN-YEAR-OLDS

Among young people aged fifteen to nineteen the facts on suicide are staggering: for every death by drowning there are three suicides; for every three murders, four suicides occur; and for every two teenagers who die in auto accidents, one suicide is reported.

According to the National Center for Health Statistics (1990), 902 children aged fifteen to nineteen and more than 3,000 young adults between twenty and twenty-four years of age committed suicide in 1987. These depressing figures (keeping in mind that these are just the *reported* suicides) have made suicide the second leading cause of death in both age groups. The death rate is about 10 per 100,000 in the population for fifteen- to nineteen-year-olds and 15 in twenty- to twenty-four-year-olds. The death toll from suicide for males is five times higher than that for females, and the suicide rate for white males is higher than for any other racial group (Miller et al., 1986).

The method of choice in most of these suicides is some type of firearm or handgun. In fact, it is the chief method used in all three groups—from those aged five to twenty-four. The second most popular method for committing suicide is some form of suffocation, whether it be hanging or strangulation. The third ranking method of committing suicide in these age categories is by the inhalation of gases and vapors (e.g., carbon monoxide poisoning).

A fellow nurse told me about a fifteen-year-old rape victim she had treated. The young woman had been sodomized by her boyfriend's father. She was, of course, devastated by the experience and received counseling after the rape. However, she was also subjected to considerable pressure from her small community to withdraw the charges against the man in question. A short time after the incident, she committed suicide with a shotgun.

A nurse with whom I worked had a son who committed suicide at the age of fourteen. Trouble with peers, his parents' divorce, and the lack of counseling when it was needed most seemed to trigger the emotions that resulted in this suicide. The child hanged himself in his bedroom.

I have discussed the topic of suicide with both my teenage son and daughter and various of their friends. Although none of them have considered it an alternative to confronting the many problems and pressures faced by young people their age, they have encountered friends who have given serious thought to ending their own lives. One friend told me that her boyfriend has attempted suicide with drugs on several occasions. Each time he was treated and released from the hospital but has never returned for follow-up counseling. One young man told me about a male friend of his who apparently committed suicide by strangulation, but he's not sure that it was intentional. Apparently, the victim had heard that by compressing the arteries in his neck with a tie or any similar binding while masturbating, the pleasure associated with orgasm would be even greater. The victim had tried this several times before his death, so although he was ultimately thought to have committed suicide, it might simply have been a case of having carried a form of erotic stimulation too far.

SUMMARY

Suicide is a deadly menace in the fifteen-to-nineteen age range. The risks are even more pronounced in college students, among whom suicide is the second leading cause of death. However, even children five years of age and up are at risk. Our society asks a lot of its children. They have inherited a world infinitely more complex and stressful than that of their parents. We need to find ways to help them cope while we try to understand the social, emotional, and physical pressures that appear to them overpowering and at times insurmountable. Adults have to know the warning signs. Parents, teachers, friends, and others have to be attuned to the signals and move to help as soon as possible. We also have to teach children to recognize their suicidal thoughts and show them how to seek help. As parents we must realize the impact of suicide on the victim's siblings and friends and be prepared to move quickly to prevent similar action on their part. It is not uncommon for communities to be rocked by several teen suicides following one after another.

While discussing the topic of teen suicide with a colleague of mine, I was told the story of a suicide that had occurred at her child's high school. Apparently, the suicide victim was not very popular; in fact, the individual was the object of teasing and a great many jokes. However, when the child took her own life, all of the students at the school went to the funeral and brought a rose to place on the casket.

When my colleague talked to her own child and a few of her friends about their actions, she was not surprised to find that there was a certain amount of guilt about the suicide. What did surprise her was the students' perception that the victim was getting a great deal of attention as a result of her lethal act. These surviving students were enthralled by this attention and their part in the activities following her death. Their perception of this tragedy has implications for the clustering of suicides in this age group.

The reasons and warning signals for suicide are fairly clear. However, we are not always as sensitive as we should be to the clues. We must become aware and tuned in to potential victims. But more must be done to deal with the impact of suicide on those youngsters close to the victim so that these tragic circumstances do not spread like a virus throughout the community.

6

Homicide

INTRODUCTION

Homicide as a result of child abuse continues to be a leading cause of death in children of all ages. Child maltreatment accounts for about twenty-four thousand injuries (Hawkins, 1986) and approximately one thousand to twelve hundred children's deaths per year (Miller et al., 1986). We know that child abusers tend to have been abused children themselves, so an emerging repetitive and vicious cycle is often exposed. Many times the abuse goes undetected by health-care workers and other adults near the child. All too often the abuser is a parent or adult in the household who denies that a problem exists or resists the need for psychological help. In such cases, the children risk serious physical injury or even death. New and tougher laws requiring specific health-care workers to report suspected child abuse are in place in many areas and required educational programs have been developed to help medical professionals recognize the earliest signs of abuse.

As children become teenagers, they can still be victims of violence, but now the perpetrators tend to be acquaintances rather than parents. This teenage violence, of special concern to those living in our inner cities, may lead to homicide and appears to be related to drugs, alcohol, and gang-type activities. Many reports rank murder or homicide as the third leading cause of death in teenagers who live in major cities (Testa and Wulczyn, 1980). This homicide rate has doubled since the 1950s.

The fact that murder may be the third leading cause of death in teenagers who live in major urban areas makes us realize the full impact of drugs and gang-related activities on our youth. In the lobby of one Los Angeles school there hangs a student-made plaque listing the names of five hundred friends, relatives, and neighbors who have died. Almost 80 percent of these deaths were related to gang activities. We need to attack the conditions that cultivate and perpetuate this violence. Gangs thrive in poor neighborhoods. Drugs and related activities exist everywhere. "Just say no" campaigns are not enough. Cocaine and its variations, most particularly crack and ice, and all the other illegal drugs need to be eradicated to stop the violence. And let us not forget anabolic steroids: one in fifteen young Americans uses them. Most of these steroids are obtained illegally on the black market. Users tend to be athletes who want to look good and perform better in sports. However, these drugs can produce serious physical conditions, such as heart problems, with long-term use. They also can cause depression and suicidal behavior if the child stops taking them suddenly. Children start taking steroids as early as fifteen or even younger in some cases (*U.S. News and World Report,* December 26, 1988). We need to look at the environment and values of our children where these drugs are commonplace and acceptable. Drugs must be attacked at their source to save our children.

HOMICIDE AND ABUSE IN INFANTS

According to the National Center for Health Statistics (1990), 273 infants under the age of one year were the victims of homicide in 1987. The overall homicide rate was slightly higher for males than for females (8 male and 6.4 female deaths per 100,000 in the population). The death rate for African-American children is three to four times higher than for white children of the same age. The assault on these infants was usually brought on by the physical abuse of another person rather than being the result of a weapon. Of the 273 cases of homicide involving infant victims, 256 were directly related to abuse (NCHS, 1990).

As a nurse, I have seen infants who have been battered and bruised. Most often the abuser in such cases is a woman; however, when the abuse results in death, the father or a live-in boyfriend is usually involved (Hawkins, 1986). But make no mistake, *anyone can be an abuser.* The experience of a neighbor of mine will serve as a case in point. For the sake of anonymity, I'll call her Jane.

Several years ago, when Jane's child was just a baby, she had a young teenage girl who would watch the child when she and her husband would go out for the evening. This babysitter was the daughter of a neighbor with whom she had become friends. On one occasion, the couple had left for the theater, but on their way my friend realized that she had forgotten the tickets, so they returned home to get them. As Jane walked to the door, she heard her infant's muffled screaming. She rushed to the door and ran in the direction of her baby's cries. In the kitchen she found the child crying in its highchair. The babysitter, not hearing the mother's approach, slapped the infant across the face. Jane was soon able to connect this abusive behavior to the red marks or small bruises she had noticed on the child's body after the sitter had watched the baby. These had been explained away as the result of an accident with a toy or some other plaything.

On another occasion, a small infant had been left with a neighbor while its parents attended an afternoon wedding. Upon returning home, the parents had to rush the child to an emergency room. The neighbor had placed the infant outside in her backyard in a playpen that had been exposed to direct summer sun. The baby had sustained terrible burns on his body and was severely dehydrated. Several of the burns were so severe that they required substantial medical therapy. When the neighbor was questioned, she stated that she had put the baby outside because the child would not stop crying and she couldn't get anything done around the house.

As a nurse, it always amazed me how parents could hurt or neglect their own children. I have seen babies with burns, fractures, and other injuries that were unmistakably inflicted by parents, who would attempt to explain away these injuries or tell the medical staff that they were just disciplining the children. However, it is no longer as easy to offer such excuses because health-care providers have become better informed; besides, these abusive episodes happen too frequently to escape notice.

HOMICIDE AND ABUSE IN CHILDREN

Among youngsters aged one to fourteen, homicide most often strikes children between the ages of one and two years. Again, the death rate is lowest for whites and highest for African-Americans. Under the age of one, the death rate for males exceeds that for females; but from one to fourteen years of age, homicide deaths among African-American females outpaces the figures for males of the same racial background. The homicide rate for white females remains equal to or lower than that for white males, at least until four years of age when it becomes slightly higher and remains so until age fourteen. The main method utilized in the deaths of these children is some form of physical assault not involving traditional lethal weapons such as guns or knives (NCHS, 1990). In 1987, 741 children who died as a result of homicide were in the one-to-fourteen-year age category (NCHS, 1990). According to independent sources, these deaths were the direct result of physical abuse by adults (Hawkins, 1986). In a few cases the death was not abuse related or the assailant was not an adult.

In general, the majority of homicides in this age category are caused by physical assault (over 400 cases in 1987). As the child gets older, the risk of homicide from assault with a handgun or firearm increases. To illustrate, between the ages of one and five, 41 children died by this means. However, from age six to fourteen, deaths increased to well over 200 (NCHS, 1990). The remaining homicides in this age category were committed with a cutting or piercing instrument. Homicide is the sixth leading cause of death in children one to fourteen years of age (NCHS, 1990).

Many children grow up in family situations where the line between discipline and abuse is thin indeed. Take, for example, the case of a four-year-old boy who had broken some valuable Christmas ornaments. A relative made him walk barefoot on the broken glass so that he would never again touch them. Or consider the father who would hit baseballs as hard as he could at his own eight-year-old son so that the boy would not be a "sissy" and would catch the baseball properly. The same man also beat his four-year-old daughter with a wooden rake because she was crying "too loud." Eventually a relative intervened to stop this abuse.

Violence between parents can often spill over to involve young children, causing injury and even death. One man told me that when he was a child of seven, his parents began arguing one evening over dinner, at which point dishes began to fly. The father then brutally beat the mother. The children were threatened, hit with fists, and thrown about during this argument. They ultimately ran out into the night seeking cover. On another occasion, when this man was a bit older, he actually had to threaten his father at knife-point to make him stop beating his mother and to allow himself and his mother to leave the house safely.

Another unnerving story was related to me by a middle-aged man whom I'll name Dick. He did not remember the events directly but was made aware of them by his father when he was well advanced into manhood. Dick has spent most of his life in therapy and has occasionally been hospitalized for severe depression. His father, a rather quiet and remote man, grew closer to his son during late adolescence and adulthood, especially after he and Dick's mother were divorced while Dick was a toddler. It took many years for the father to open up about his son's early childhood. Dick does not remember many of the events that took place during long periods of his early life. This inability to recall has interfered to some extent with his counseling therapy.

The father relayed several compelling episodes in his son's toddler years, all of which began to shed light on Dick's childhood and the legacy of emotional and physical abuse that may have helped to create his mental deterioration seen later in young adulthood. Dick obviously has forgotten or repressed many of these memories.

His father told him that early in his marriage, Dick's mother began to have affairs with other men. Occasionally, she would bring them home while he worked nights. Dick and his siblings were exposed to a variety of strange men who had sexual relations with their mother while they were in the house. She would also leave these young children alone in the house when she would go out for dates at night.

One night, she wanted to leave and no one was home but two-year-old Dick. Apparently, she knew she would be out all night and had no one to keep an eye on her son. So she put him to bed in the late afternoon and tied him down in his crib so that he could not move. Dick may have slept for a while, but when he awoke there was no one around and it could have been dark. No one will ever know what really happened, but his mother never returned until the following morning. In the meantime, when Dick's father returned home around midnight, he found the house empty. Dick's siblings were with a neighbor and obviously the mother wasn't present. Dick's father, unaware, went from room to room looking for them. When he came into Dick's room, he was horrified to find his son tied in his crib, Dick's tear-streaked face frozen in a silent scream, his arms firmly fixed alongside his face while he lay in his own urine and feces. Dick's father untied his son, cleaned him up, held him, and rocked him. He sang to him, talked to him, and after a few hours, Dick began to respond.

His father confronted the mother, but never pursued it further. They divorced a few years after this, but because of the lack of documentation regarding this abuse, the father never conveyed the incident to the court, so the mother gained custody of her son. The father has never been able to understand why she wanted custody, since the pattern of neglect and physical abuse continued—she always viewed Dick as an imposition. Because of his horror and shame at what had happened to his son, Dick's father never told anyone. Thus, Dick never knew until he was an adult and began to try to reconstruct his childhood during therapy. His father was very resistant at first but eventually opened up.

Over the years, during his brief visitation periods, Dick's father would notice welts and bruises on his son's face and body. Regrettably, the father contributed to this situation in his own way by never confronting the situation legally. In Dick's school-age years, his mother gave him to his father because she had remarried by then and Dick's stepfather was abusive, an alcoholic, and didn't like the little boy.

Dick remembers very little of what his childhood was like. He has no memories before age eleven, except those related to school events during this period. Recently, he has had other more traumatic events come back to his conscious memory. Over a period of ten years, he has put these sparse memories together. He remembers some of the physical abuse, but what he remembers most is the mental abuse. Dick was constantly told he was worthless and unwanted, and when his parents were drunk, the stepfather would beat the mother and then turn on him. The beatings stopped when Dick went to live with his father. Eventually, he was forced to return to the mother. Apparently, she did not want Dick's father to have permanent custody of the child—for financial reasons. In court, the father failed to win custody. Dick was never brought to court, the judge believing that a child should always be with its natural mother, and she still had legal custody. However, by then the physical abuse stopped because Dick had grown up and the stepfather had since died. The mental berating continued, however, until adulthood. During college Dick tried to commit suicide; it was then that the ravages of depression began to surface.

When I met Dick, counseling sessions had largely helped him to resolve these issues in his past. However, he wanted me to include his story because he believes children are too vulnerable to abusive parents and adults. Even though he didn't die as a result of this abuse, he feels that a part of him is lost forever and that he has endured a lifetime of depression and suicidal thoughts. He believes people can die inside, especially children!

None of these incidents resulted in death but, again, they demonstrate how abuse and discipline are easily confused or misinterpreted and how the battering of a woman by her spouse or male live-in lover can seriously threaten a child's safety. In many instances the battering of wives involves the abuse of children as well (Children's Defense Fund, 1989). Even though these victims may not die, they will always be emotionally scarred. Years later they can barely talk about these events without a great deal of trauma and fear.

78   Our Children Are Dying

TEENAGERS AND HOMICIDE

In 1987, as previously noted, 741 children between one and fourteen years of age died as a result of homicide (NCHS, 1990). In addition, there was a dramatic increase in the number of homicides in fifteen to nineteen-year-olds. In the latter age group, 1,838 teen homicide victims were reported. The greatest proportion of these homicides among the teenagers resulted from assault with some type of firearm (handgun, rifle, shotgun): over 1,300 cases in all. The second most prevalent method of homicide was assault with a cutting, piercing, or unspecified instrument.

Reflecting on the National Adolescent Study Health Survey (1987), discussed early in this book (see chapter 1), it will be recalled that a fairly large number of students had been threatened or attacked by peers as early as the eighth grade. These statistics demonstrate how very dangerous some of our neighborhoods are for our teenage children. In this fifteen-to nineteen-year-old age group, males are more often victims of homicide than females, and the death rate for African-American males is proportionately higher than for any other group in this age bracket (NCHS, 1990).

SUMMARY

The rate at which violent death is affecting our children has reached epidemic proportions. Child abuse has become a factor that no longer discriminates on the bases of race, religion, socioeconomic class, or education. Battered children can be found anywhere. We must examine ways to deal effectively with parental and adult abuse. Our system of monitoring seems to have more and more difficulty coping with the enormity of this problem. Of all the ways death claims the youth of America, the problem of parental abuse is the cruelest. Our children should be protected; why then are they so often the victims of those who gave them life? How can society move to change this emerging ruthless pattern? What we are doing doesn't seem to be working. We need to be better able to identify abusers and to help them, while at the same time ensuring the safety of our children.

In teenagers, the evidence demonstrates that homicide is indeed a major cause of death. It ranks third among fifteen- to nineteen-year-olds. Gang activities and drugs are thought to be major factors in these deaths.

Traditionally, teenagers from turbulent, stressful homes often run away. In some cases, they have been victims of physical, emotional, and/or sexual abuse. As a result, once away from the protection of home, they are at the mercy of the "streets" and often fall victim to violence, exploitation, and even death (Hawkins, 1986).

Part Two

The View from the Trenches

7

The Experts Speak Out

Part One focused on a detailed discussion of the risks facing today's youth and the challenge to be met by parents and concerned adults. It is abundantly clear that the dangers confronting our nation's children are considerable, but we are not without weapons in the fight to save the lives of countless young people. Social service agencies on the federal, state, and local levels exist to safeguard those of our children whose lives are jeopardized in ways that bring substantial numbers of them under the custodial care of specific agencies. Unfortunately, these protective services and oversight agencies exist through funding provided by the various levels of government. For many organizations their mission can be greatly modified by a lack of funding or other available support. In some instances, there may be significant gaps in the services provided by the different agencies created to support children. Again, by looking at what agencies do and where the gaps exist, we may be able to prevent innocent children from falling through the cracks.

The point of this discussion is not to attack any one particular agency because, as all who work in the field of child welfare know and agree, the major line of defense against childhood death is composed of thoughtful, caring, and concerned parents and adults. For instance, accidents occur when children are close to home. Therefore, various child welfare agencies can provide support, but they can never replace the safety of a good home with caring parents. Different agencies move in to protect children who are at risk if parents are not providing that protection or are harming the children.

As a nation, we should be far more concerned with parenting and with teaching people how to improve their skills in that all-important role. On the other hand, we also have to be able to intervene effectively when any problems related to parenting or adult supervision occur. If some in our society who do not fulfill their parental obligations toward their children consciously choose not to live up to their legal and moral responsibilities, society's concerned citizens must do whatever they can to protect these youngsters. Of course, we also acknowledge the fact that some parents want very much to do a good job but do not have the resources, knowledge, and or emotional support to succeed.

In this chapter we are going to look more closely at the available support systems to determine their effectiveness. Instead of running through a complete list of organizations focusing on the responsibilities of each, it seemed that much more could be gained by listening to the dedicated men and women who are on the front lines everyday. It is they who can offer a fresh insight into how parents can start doing a better job, what must be done when they don't, and how to make the system more responsive to the needs of all children.

I conducted a series of four interviews with experts representing various social-service programs and agencies. What follows are synopses of these interviews. To protect the identities of the interviewees, each has been given a fictitious name.

"PAUL"

My first interview was with "Paul," the director of community health programs for a hospital, who also has a great deal of experience in discharge planning (helping patients make the transition from hospital to home) and in nursing. According to Paul, health care has become very complex in recent years, and access for poor people is difficult at best. Many who cannot afford health insurance or have limited coverage discover that preventive health care is often beyond their grasp. They can get emergency care, but often not before an illness has become a major—sometimes life or death—problem.

Poor parents are eligible for Medicaid health benefits, but many physicians limit the number of such patients they will accept. If a mother lacks health insurance or is dependent on Medicaid, she may not be eligible for certain types of health care or has limited access because of the amount Medicaid will reimburse for specific services. To help address these deficiencies, Paul's hospital initiated a telephone line to assist people in the community to find needed services and to provide guidance on issues related to health care. Because many young families don't have adequate health care coverage or are ill-informed, their children often suffer.

Another factor that Paul isolated as having a significant impact on child welfare and the untimely death of infants is the increasing rate of teenage pregnancy. These young women are often emotionally unprepared for the harsh realities of child-rearing. Usually they have not used any birth control method to prevent the pregnancy. There is rarely much education available to them on a regular basis regarding pregnancy. In an attempt to hide or deny the pregnancy, these frightened young people frequently do not seek help until the late stages—the last couple of months. Moreover, the babies of teenage mothers are many times neglected and abused unless another supportive, more mature adult is available to help with child care. Unfortunately, child abuse is not confined to one social class or ethnic group; it pervades all segments of society. As we have seen, the incidents of child abuse are on the rise and the medical as well as social-work systems are losing their ability to intervene effectively to help parents modify their abusive tendencies while simultaneously protecting the vulnerable child.

In summary, Paul believes that lack of access to health care, the increasing number of teenage pregnancies, and the rising incidence of child abuse are major contributors to the death of our children. He offers these recommendations for parents:

1. Obtain good prenatal care. Consult the local social services agency to determine what programs are available in the community for pregnant mothers to get prenatal care if they can't afford it or do not have health insurance.

2. Attend classes that teach techniques of effective parenting.

3. Seek counseling for abusive tendencies.

4. Promptly report suspected child abuse to the proper authorities.

5. Educate teenagers regarding safe sex and contraception. Make sure teens are aware of effective birth control methods and are knowledgeable about where they can get advice and support.

For concerned citizens Paul has this advice:

1. Encourage free or low-cost community education services through local schools, hospitals, and churches to conduct parent training

programs such as Parent Effectiveness Training or specific classes on selected aspects of parenting or child-rearing techniques.

2. Try to encourage local hospitals and clinics to conduct free classes for young mothers on infant care.

3. Encourage local legislators to allocate funds for health care services to those populations who cannot afford them.

4. Make sure that there are community self-help programs and support groups for child abusers.

5. Contribute time, effort, and/or money to organizations that help fill the gaps in community services to these high-risk groups.

6. Examine the services available to teens in terms of sex education, birth control, and pregnancy. Look at access and availability.

"CLARA"

My second interview was with a former case worker for a social-service agency. Clara is a very verbal, assertive, and forthright individual with an active, honest knowledge and interest in underprivileged populations. In fact she left social services to assume another position in a related child-welfare program because she had difficulty coping over a long period of time with the large number of abuse cases she handled in social services. She felt frustrated that her efforts to reach out and help these children were not more successful. Clara is an active member of an inner city African-American church and has personal and professional experience with this cultural group.

I asked her to share with me some of this first-hand knowledge and experience. For her protection and that of her former clients, this information will be presented in general terms rather than as individual cases.

The primary factor that Clara feels has a significant negative impact on services provided for children is the lack of public input with regard to the delivery of specific services in communities. Some of the programs that are supposedly available are not readily accessible using public transportation, and often their hours of availability are so limited that many people who need the services or could benefit from them give up trying to make use of them. Other services or programs are not always sensitive to the real needs of the community so they are both underutilized and ineffective. Clara also says that some community programs have a high turnover of volunteers or employees so that services are inconsistent and sometimes of poor quality. She gives as an example an afterschool educational and meal program that provided tutoring and free meals to underprivileged children. The volunteers for the tutoring component dwindled to zero. Eventually the children came for the meals and wrote and played on the blackboard without the benefit of any educational program. She believed that the combination of limited funds and the absence of trained volunteers to conduct the education programing severely crippled this service, which was otherwise well-received in the particular community. Therefore, according to Clara, programs that directly benefit some inner-city families may be inaccessible, poorly staffed, and inadequately funded, making services inconsistent, or they do not meet the specific needs of the population for whom they were designed.

As she spoke, I recalled Nancy Milo's book titled *9226 Kercheval Street,* which discusses the development and operation of a storefront community health center in Detroit's inner city. One of the major factors that made the clinic successful was substantial neighborhood input and consideration of the needs of the population it was supposed to serve. Clara's point is well taken: services must fit the client's needs and their culture. Specific programs also need to be consistent and predictable in the type and quality of services they provide.

Clara and I went on to discuss the unfortunate death of children and the factors that she thought aggravated the increased incidence of child fatalities. Her vast experience with social services became evident as she carefully delineated these factors.

Like Paul, Clara considers teenage pregnancy to be a major element contributing to the high infant mortality rate in the U.S. population. The poor prenatal care received by these girls, their exposure to drugs and alcohol during pregnancy, and their lack of knowledge about infant care combine to produce many low-birth-weight babies who are not healthy or have serious defects at birth. These infants do not receive adequate health care in their first crucial months even if they survive birth. Although she was not sure about accessibility to prenatal care, Clara did know that many of these young girls were well advanced into their pregnancies before they received any care at all. She felt sure that teens deny the pregnancy or are uneducated regarding their options. Clara also was of the mind that our society tends to glamorize sex and at times even single parenthood. Many of the celebrities teens look up to have openly elected single parenthood.

As for child-care or medical services for infants, Clara stated that these were quite limited and difficult to obtain if the parent was on Medicaid or had no health insurance. She cited cutbacks in government funding as a reason for this limitation and emphasized that reduced expenditures had a tremendous impact on infant health care. Medical care is virtually nonexistent for many of our poorer citizens these days. She recounted the story of one young mother who took her sick infant to the emergency room of a hospital. The young mother told the staff of the emergency room that she was on Medicaid but did not have her card with her, so they made her go home and get it. Lacking a car, she had to use public transportation to get back and forth—precious time that could have resulted in her child's death. According to Clara, hospitals are under tremendous pressure to show a profit; therefore some services to the poor and underprivileged are difficult to obtain or nonexistent.

Clara also stated that young teenagers with a child do not have access to good child care. If parents don't agree to help, these new parents end up taking care of their children themselves. As a result, the teens do not finish school, which severely limits their job opportunities. Many times they become bored with the child and the total commitment of their time to the new infant. It is not at all uncommon for them to leave the infant (or child) alone at times or place the youngster in the hands of anyone who will babysit free of charge. More often than not such actions place the children in grave danger.

Child abuse in this less affluent population is a frequent occurrence. In many of the cases of infant deaths related to child abuse, Clara discovered a young, unmarried mother who was struggling with inadequate alternatives for child care. Two deaths were the direct result of live-in boyfriends who beat the infants to death. Having a live-in helps with the rent and expenses as well as child care, and it's a frequent alternative for many young women. But Clara considers it a hidden danger for both infants and young children.

She found that in some neighborhoods mothers who were receiving public assistance funds (low-income women with children who meet requirements) did not get enough money to make ends meet. If these women were employed and made over a certain dollar amount, they were considered ineligible for food stamps and other aid programs. Rather than risk reduced aid, many decided not to work. Some turn to prostitution or to selling drugs as a way of making unreported extra money. However, as Clara states, the children in these homes suffer immeasurably and are exposed to many unsavory characters who threaten their welfare. Child abuse and neglect prevail in this atmosphere of uncertainty.

Another problem mentioned by Clara is that in child-abuse cases the youngsters often remain in the home while charges against the parents are pending. Unless the danger to the children is great enough to warrant immediate removal from the home, they are kept in a situation that is potentially abusive and dangerous. In one example she cited, a teacher reported a potential child-abuse case during school hours. The child had been beaten with a belt; numerous welts and cuts were evident on the boy's back. The youngster left school to return home, and it was twenty-four hours before anyone from a child welfare agency went to the home to investigate.

As for treatment of those who abuse their children, it is limited and sporadic. A key hurdle, Clara believes, is getting parents to admit the abuse. They try generally to cover it up and are reluctant to seek help for their abusive tendencies. The system to deal with the problem is inadequate and the strategies for helping the child as well as the parents are insufficient and inconsistent. Parents' rights often take precedence over the child's. Case loads are huge and case workers "burn out" quickly. It is not uncommon for investigators to be personally threatened. Clara finally left her job because she could no longer cope with the frustration.

In cases where a child was killed, abuse had been suspected by neighbors or others but had been inadequately reported or ignored entirely. Clara indicates that reporting abuse is no easy matter; people who do report it ultimately are reluctant to testify in court, so they prefer to remain anonymous. Clara believes that it is easier to prove abuse in lower-income families. When cases involve more affluent parents, it tends to be difficult to document and easier for the parents to cover up the whole thing. It is difficult to provide support or follow-up in such cases.

In many child-abuse cases, the mother has also been "battered." The woman may be reluctant to report this because of the effects on her relationship with the boyfriend or spouse. It's an extremely frustrating situation for case workers because even after the woman seeks help and has the man arrested, she often goes back to him whereupon the cycle of battering and abuse begins again. Unfortunately, the children are often physically and emotionally injured. The harm may last a lifetime.

On the subject of teenage deaths, Clara points out that although crisis services are available for suicidal children, parents and other adults may not pick up on symptoms soon enough. A child often does not get help until a suicide attempt has been made. At that point, it is sometimes too late. Clara feels that suicide is chiefly a disease of white middle-class males. Their problems did not stem from poverty but from affluence. Many of these middle-class kids have money but little parental supervision and guidance. The resulting emotional problems then get out of hand. She also believes that some accidental deaths among teenagers may really be suicide attempts or the result of a "death wish" that manifests itself in excessive risk-taking. Recognizing suicidal tendencies is more of a problem than obtaining treatment. Parents or other adults are simply not aware of the danger signals and so they often react too late.

In regard to alcohol and drugs, Clara thinks these are overwhelming problems affecting all social classes across the board. However, the availability of drugs and the dangers associated with their sale are problems that surface more in an urban than a suburban setting. She believes that middle-class teenagers use drugs as a method of entertainment, whereas poor youths get involved with, use, and sell drugs to escape poverty. The young feed on the young. They make money by selling drugs to other kids.

"Gate houses" for the making and sale of illicit drugs are more often in the inner city, where abandoned houses and buildings are readily available. In one neighborhood where Clara observed a "drug house" operating, it was not at all uncommon for the house to get raided periodically by the police. But once the raid was over, the "tenants" would return. One house had even been refurbished with urban redevelopment funds. It was then rented by "drug thugs."

Illegal drugs are readily available. Clara told me about one instance in which she was following up on a referral. She rang the bell and identified herself. The people in the house actually tried to sell her drugs because they believed she was using her name and title as a cover to buy them. Once she verified her identification, they threatened her life.

Another side effect of our drug-oriented society, according to Clara, is the rapid increase in the number of "crack babies"—children born of cocaine-addicted mothers. In many instances, pregnant women are jailed instead of treated for their addiction; therefore, they tend to avoid the system rather than seeking help for themselves and their unborn children. Clara saw evidence that even young children were being swept up in the drug culture. There is very little ongoing education for inner-city children regarding drugs and alcohol and little to counter the excitement, glamour, and profit that young kids from poor backgrounds find so fascinating about "dealing." And, of course, there is also the thrill-seeking middle- and upper-class young people who can afford the recreational drug environment.

In summary, the problems outlined by Clara are evidenced throughout this volume. The problems center around:

1. the increase in teenage pregnancies and inadequate care during pregnancy;

2. inadequate monitoring and intervention in cases of child abuse and neglect;

3. the lack of funds to provide services to needy groups and the lack of sensitivity of existing services to the cultural and ethnic populations they serve;

4. the decreasing availability of health care and child care to the populations whose members need them most;

5. the availability of and dangers associated with illegal drugs as well as the lack of positive role models who could help steer young people away from drug and alcohol use;

6. and poverty and discrimination: the former breeds many of the ills that threaten children, while the latter threatens to create a permanent underclass.

After discussing the problems that serve to create an environment antagonistic to child welfare, I asked Clara what she thought parents and citizens could do to help reduce preventable childhood death. I especially wanted her to address the needs of African-Americans and other ethnic minorities, in addition to Caucasian children, because of her ethnic and cultural heritage as well as her experience. Since the incidence of childhood death is a much bigger problem in the African-American community, it seemed sensible to address it specifically. For parents of children in this high-risk population Clara offers the following recommendations:

1. Teach young women early about the necessity of birth control. Make sure they get the information and contraceptive materials they need to prevent pregnancy. Don't assume that because a woman is young, she's not sexually active. Don't leave sex education to someone else. It may or may not be provided, but if young girls are learning from friends, the information will be grossly inadequate.

2. Likewise, educate your sons about sex. Reinforce the need to use condoms, not only to ensure safe sex (avoiding sexually transmitted diseases) but to avoid pregnancy.

3. Educate children *early* to the dangers of drugs and alcohol.

4. Be as involved as you can with your child's school. Know your child's teachers and counselors. Make sure that programs designed to educate about drugs and alcohol are in place.

5. Be aware of the community resources available to your child and use them to your best advantage.

6. Take the time to get to know your children *and* their friends. Listen to them and be especially sensitive to possible problems. Make your children feel good about themselves; reward their accomplishments.

7. If you must leave your children in someone else's charge, make sure that the person who cares for them is responsible and caring. If your child is alone, make sure he or she has someone to go to or call if help is needed.

8. Be politically active and aware on behalf of your children. Be aware of a politician's record with regard to child-welfare issues. Vote accordingly!

Clara feels some programs or approaches on the community level would be helpful. Here are some of her suggestions:

1. Make child care available in schools so teenage mothers can finish high school.

2. Provide adult-education classes where free or low-cost child care is available. Mothers can then obtain training without the difficulties inherent in finding child care.

3. Increase accessibility to child care for the poor. Funding cutbacks have severely reduced this service. Increased accessibility to health care in general for the poor would be a great benefit.

4. Support efforts to continue and increase funding for the Head Start Program.* It's a good program and it makes a difference. Training for parents should coincide with this program so that they can obtain a high-school equivalency diploma or enroll in effective parenting classes. Programs should be available for unskilled young men who have fathered children, thus providing them with training so they can later enter the workforce and ultimately be capable of supporting or contributing to the support of the child or children they helped create.

---

*A federal program of early childhood education which provides disadvantaged youngsters with a range of crucial services (Children's Defense Fund, 1989)

5. Work with neighbors and law enforcement agencies to force drugs out of the community (possibly through neighborhood watch programs).

6. Ensure that community organizations reinforce the schools by providing education on drugs and alcohol.

7. Make birth control and sex education available in the junior and senior high schools or make sure clinics and services are more accessible than presently is the case, especially to high-risk teenage populations.

8. Encourage legislators to revise current systems of welfare: one suggestion being to raise the amount of money a person can earn under the current child-welfare system without forfeiting a proportional amount of benefits.

9. Make local, state, and national legislators more responsive to children's issues by becoming politically active.

10. Streamline and centralize the system for reporting child abuse. Ensure that an abuse hotline is in place and easy to use. Make sure there are counseling and/or support groups for abusers as well as the abused.

"JOHN"

I next spoke with "John," a government health official whose knowledge and experience regarding child health and welfare issues spans many years.

According to John, a major problem with children's services and programs is the manner in which they are funded by the various government sources. During the Reagan administration, funding for each state was provided in the form of a block grant for maternal child services. This lump sum to the state was expected to cover all the programs and services provided to children. Since there was only one pot of money, agencies jockeyed and scrambled to compete for their fair share of the incoming funds. In many states good cooperation exists among all the state-wide children's agencies, but in some states cooperation is nonexistent. In the latter, the competition among various agencies often results in duplication and overlap of services. Many agencies do a little, but nobody can afford to do a lot for any group. This description may oversimplify a bit the inadequacies within this system of funding, but as John says, the end result of all this is that there are many agencies with similar programs that do exactly the same thing. Since there is not always a great deal of cooperation among these agencies, the recipients of social services suffer from the duplication of inadequate services.

In addition to these problems, the amount of money provided to the states for all agency programs does not increase dramatically from year to year even though the annual costs of running these programs are constantly rising. Budgets are not "indexed" for inflation, meaning they are not increased to cover the reduced buying power of the agency. Therefore, for an agency to survive it has to cut back or eliminate services to keep pace with increasing costs. This can have a serious impact on the quality and quantity of services available to children who are most in need of the available help. In addition, many agencies on the state level have large administrative structures or bureaucracies that utilize a substantial portion of the monies allocated. If the agency or organization has many levels of management, the administrative costs snowball. Since states tend to have a variety of agencies managing children's support and protective services, there are expensive administrative costs at every level. Therefore, a great deal of money is spent on managing often overlapping programs, which leaves inadequate funds for the actual implementation of these services.

Beyond the obvious deficits and mismanagement in program funding, John identifies many of the same social conditions that others have described: increasing numbers of teenage pregnancies, poverty, discrimination, ignorance, lack of good care of the mother during pregnancy, and poor nutrition produce an increasing number of low-birth-weight babies, which raises the likelihood of infant death. John also emphasizes that although we tend to highlight the problems of the poor in urban areas, we often forget how difficult it is for the rural poor to gain access to services, and they may be quite ill-informed about what is available and why they need to ensure that a mother and new infant have adequate health care. He indicates that although the amount of money provided nationwide to families via welfare may be inadequate or minimal, there are families who, because of pride or ignorance, do not obtain even this minimal aid—Medicaid, food stamps, or WIC (Women, Infants, and Children Program).

He indicates that doctors in rural areas may be few in number and widely dispersed among the population; and if they have limited the number of Medicaid patients they will accept, the rural poor may not have any available care except that found in the emergency room of the nearest hospital. This in turn increases the demand for services in our hospitals and the waiting time in these facilities.

John also cautions against blaming physicians for limiting the number of Medicaid patients they accept. The red tape involved in Medicaid reimbursement is often horrendous, and when coupled with the fact that there have been no significant increases in Medicaid's reimbursement rate during the last several years, physicians are naturally reluctant to accept this form of payment. The "nearly poor," or those who earn too much to be eligible for Medicaid and other forms of aid, are even more of a problem in that they may have no mechanism for paying a physician. In some areas, physicians have a good number of unpaid patient bills because families cannot afford to pay for services when they are provided. There are even instances of families who may barter or offer alternate forms of compensation because they simply do not have the money to pay for medical care.

John speaks of other special populations in which the infant and child death rates may be disproportionately high in relation to the rest of the population. These populations highlight that there are other factors we need to consider when examining the death of children who are hard pressed because they are far outside the mainstream of American life. Special religious communities such as the Amish, who usually will not accept any form of government aid, cannot even be reached by some public health programs. The children of migrant families, because they live on the road and lack permanency, have very little health care and often die from illnesses and injuries that go untreated. Although state or local governments may run some form of migrant clinic, these services are sparse because there is not enough funding. Additionally, because migrants are in one place for only a short time, they are not eligible for local Medicaid funding and are often unaware of the kinds of care required and/or available for their pregnant mothers, infants, and children.

Among these special groups must be added Native Americans. Their health problems may be well managed if the tribe has elected to use Indian Health Services. In some cases, the chief may elect not to have that option for his tribe. If not, the general health services available may be completely inadequate to the community's needs. The teaching of basic health practices in these circumstances may be difficult and little federal money is available to support the effort.* Some tribes may operate child-care clinics, but

---

*By treaty the Native American population of the United States falls under the jurisdiction of the federal government.

the attendance is often very poor due to a lack of understanding on the part of the mothers.

In some areas of the country there may be pockets of illegal aliens who have no access to health care and no claim to funds. Unfortunately, the children of this group suffer terribly, as do homeless families with children. John believes that the poor who live in dilapidated housing will become the homeless of the future. These homeless children have virtually no services to which they have access on a consistent basis. When we consider preventable childhood death, we should remember the needs of these oppressed and often forgotten segments of our population.

John also discusses the services available to children throughout the various age groups we've been addressing. Most programs in the United States are geared to children from infancy to about five years of age. Thereafter, the services available to school-age children and teenagers are often quite limited. Who provides primary health-care services to these groups? What kind of safety and prevention programs are available? Some school districts have excellent school health programs; however, many do not. There are significant nutritional problems with this school-age group, such as iron deficiency anemia and stunted growth. What will be the long-term effects of these nutritional deficits on their adult years? John feels that it will be far more costly in the future if we ignore problems of the present.

With regard to teenagers, John notes that in many states clinics are located in the schools to provide not only testing for pregnancy and sexually transmitted diseases but counseling as well. He feels that clinics designed for adolescents would be best able to meet the needs of teens, because there are currently very few places for them to go to get discreet health care and counseling and there is virtually no federal funding available for this type of service. In light of the trends in adolescent pregnancy and sexually transmitted disease, accessible clinics may provide a sensible solution. In any case, the services to older children and teens are inadequate under the present system. We need better youth services!

As our previous discussion demonstrated, a major problem in this country is child abuse and neglect. The present systems in place to monitor it are inadequate and the limited services available to protect children may be further depleted by the increased numbers of reported abuse cases. John believes that more childhood deaths from abuse could be prevented if the system were better funded and had additional personnel who were adequately trained and experienced to monitor these cases.

John also describes two special problems that he feels contribute to the death rate among our nation's children: both are related to pregnancy.

The first is the increasing incidence of battered pregnant women. If this violence to the pregnant mother is severe, an infant can be stillborn or otherwise become a death statistic. There is also evidence to suggest that the stress produced in these mothers by having to endure this type of harsh living condition may have additional negative effects, particularly on the developing fetuses of those women for whom the abuse has continued for a long period of time.

The second problem concerns the increased incidence of cocaine use. Mothers addicted to crack cocaine often neglect getting care during their pregnancy. In some areas, if a mother obtains medical care and tests positive for drug use, she is arrested and jailed. The arrest is a signal to other poor pregnant mothers to avoid the system altogether: a dangerous decision, since we already know that these babies are more often prone to low birth weight with serious physical problems after the birth. Therefore, the present system reinforces the fact that the mother is "bad" rather than ill and in need of counseling and prenatal care.

As we have seen, there are a great many reasons for the presence of low-birth-weight babies but these two have become more threatening of late. John notes that prenatal care for these young women is less costly than the high-tech care their babies often require once they are born. He believes that even if we did have all the systems in place, the societal problems associated with poverty would seriously impede our efforts to prevent childhood deaths.

The problems John identified can be summed up as follows:

1. The decreases in funding for adequate child-care services have seriously impeded the effort to improve child welfare and to prevent childhood illness, injury, and death.

2. Duplication and inadequate service typify the current state of child welfare delivery. A little is being done by several agencies, while high administrative costs exist for each agency involved.

3. There are increasing numbers of teenage pregnancies.

4. Many women receive inadequate prenatal care and this results in ever-increasing mortality rates among our nation's infants.

5. There are special ethnic populations who receive virtually no services or very inadequate and poorly funded ones.

6. There are very limited programs available to older children and teens.

7. Increasing numbers of women are battered during pregnancy, thus endangering the unborn children and the mothers.

8. Drug and alcohol problems are rampant among teens and children but are especially problematic in the case of pregnant women.

9. Child abuse is inadequately monitored and attempts at prevention are ineffective.

John's recommendations include the following:

1. The federal government should increase the funding available for programs aimed at children.

2. The ceiling for welfare and Medicaid payments should be increased and eligibility extended to cover health care for the nearly poor.

3. Agencies at the state level must cooperate more and eliminate duplication of services. Possibly one organization could coordinate all children's services to cut down on administrative costs and make more money available for the programs.

4. Services specifically geared to adolescents should be available.

5. School health programs should be expanded and fully supported.

6. Better access to prenatal care is needed for all expectant mothers and better prenatal and infant care education should be provided for young women of childbearing age.

7. We must have a more rational and humane approach to cocaine-addicted mothers.

"BILL"

My final interview was with "Bill," a family court judge. He frankly admitted that there were many problems with the current system of child welfare and that the failure of the system is very much in evidence in the court system.

As a judge, Bill has had more than fourteen years of experience with children and families. I asked him to describe some of the circumstances that, in his experience, contribute to the death of so many of our nation's children. Again, much like the other individuals with whom I spoke, the problems that create the circumstances conducive to increased child fatalities are really a reflection of the problems faced by our society as a whole.

One aspect that he discusses at great length is the change in the character and composition of the American family. Bill's ancestors immigrated to the United States in the early part of this century. His parents were of Polish descent. The family was very close, hard-working, survived the Depression, and eventually moved on to bigger and better things. In those days it was possible to work hard and get ahead by force of will and sheer determination. Bill's was a traditional nuclear family and all members were expected to contribute financially and emotionally to the family's survival.

According to Bill, the ethics and conduct of family business and the change in the composition and character of families have altered dramatically over the past several decades. No longer is the traditional family of mother, father, and siblings in one household the rule of thumb. Instead we have a large number of single-parent families in which the parent usually works. Dedication and hard work are not enough to survive financially in today's fast-paced, sophisticated world. One income or one parent's efforts are not enough to support a family. The costs associated with raising and educating children have skyrocketed out of control and the amount of help a family can expect from outside sources is barely enough to keep them at poverty level. Because of the "new" type of family, both children and parents experience more stress and pressure. Bill also feels that in these single-parent situations, some fathers have had very little accountability for paying any or even minimal support.

In addition, Bill feels that many of our society's more traditional values have changed. Drugs and alcohol are glamorized. Parents are hard-pressed to counteract the powerful effect of media and peers. We have also become a society that promotes promiscuity. Children are forced to make decisions early about these situations and in some cases this pressure puts them in great danger. Bill feels that movies, television, and contemporary music emphasize violence: he cites various cases in which young people appear before him and talk about how some of these influences have encouraged them to cross over the line from right to wrong. Children of all ages have become potential victims.

Bill and I talked a great deal about children who get into trouble at home, at school, or have a brush with the law. Because of repeated behavioral problems, these children often become classified as "PINS" (persons in need of supervision). Such children come to family court because the parents cannot handle their repeated problems; therefore, the court intervenes. The family court is responsible for determining ways in which the child and family can be helped. As part of this determination, an investigation into the family and the child's circumstances is conducted. Included in this investigation are psychological or psychiatric reports, social-work reports, and other types of information regarding the family. Depending on the problems and the circumstances, the child can be placed in a variety of settings. Some environments are provided for children with emotional and psychological problems. These young people often display very aggressive behavior toward the parent(s), who can no longer cope with their child's lack of response to discipline and guidance. The child is placed in an institution where counseling and schooling are provided and remains there until the problems can be solved.

Still other children may have repeated run-ins with the law. The problem of repeat offenders dictates that the environment be secure and structured to protect the child as well as society. Once the young person is sixteen, he or she can be designated as a juvenile delinquent if the crimes and circumstances warrant this and be placed in a facility specifically for juveniles who have committed criminal acts. With increasing frequency, however, young people are being placed in the adult prison system if the crime is particularly violent and it is determined that the individual is a genuine threat to society.

When asked if he thought any of the above options had a real impact on the future of these children, Bill voiced the opinion that the interventions for "PINS" were adequate and often helpful to both parent and child. As children become more and more involved with the law, the reduced availability of resources render the impact on behavior change much less pronounced. These early brushes with the law and placement in a secure, structured facility do not always act as a deterrent to criminal activity as the child grows to adulthood. As for placing youngsters in adult prisons, Bill thinks this option doesn't help anyone. However, our judicial system has a great deal of difficulty with this position. Some of the crimes committed by these youngsters are so violent that our juvenile system of incarceration would inadequately protect society from these offenders. They are in essence so dangerous that the threat of their committing further violence on society overrides the concern for their protection as children or minors. Our system, according to Bill, is reactive when it should be "proactive." We should be addressing the societal problems that combine to create an environment capable of producing criminals. We should be working with younger children to engender good moral behavior and values. We should educate children and ensure that our schools adequately prepare our young people for life. Our country has to help parents financially so they in turn can provide their children with the type of home environment that we know reduces crime. Waiting until our children become involved in crime is just too late. Once they are in the juvenile system the chances of beating the obstacles are decidedly less.

Bill recalled one situation in which a teenager had committed manslaughter. The child was placed in a secure and structured facility for a period of one year. He threatened to kill Bill when he got out, and then his detention was extended. During the total time he was detained, he received counseling. Several years thereafter, he did come to see the judge, but instead of threatening him, the young man thanked Bill. At that point, he was attending school and was planning to work with troubled children once he· finished his schooling. Unfortunately, this young man is the exception rather than the rule.

Generally, our system as it presently exists does not deter young people from committing or repeating unlawful acts. The court-authorized evaluations consider the many obstacles facing the young person, thus making it easy to determine where things go wrong in the child's life. The problems a child faces can program him or her for a life in the criminal-justice system, possibly leading to violence and even death. Very few young people who appear before Bill have had a good family life. Most suffer from a lack of self-esteem, and many have been the victims of violence and abuse as youngsters. An alarming number go on to become fatalities at a young age.

The judge also talked about the drug epidemic and the crime and violence associated with it. Drugs are not only responsible for many of our children turning to lives of crime but also for increasing numbers of teenage homicides and suicides. Young teens who become involved with illegal drugs often commit a variety of crimes to obtain the money needed to maintain their drug habits. These young people may even begin to deal drugs as a way of meeting their own drug needs and to make extra money. When they get to this point, Bill believes they run a grave risk of either becoming victims of violence or dying from a drug overdose.

Another area of concern, in his opinion, is the emergence of satanic cults which promote violence, suicide, and death among their members. Bill believes that in some communities these cults are responsible for cluster suicides and ritualistic teenage murders. He recalls one young girl who had appeared before him in a case that had definite cult overtones. On numerous occasions, the girl had demonstrated incorrigible behavior, and Bill wanted to place her in a facility for disturbed and troubled youth.

However, she pleaded to stay at home and was therefore placed on probation and allowed to return to the family environment, but only after she agreed to avoid a group of friends who were thought to be an unsavory influence. These friends had involved the girl in a variety of activities that worried her mother and had resulted in repeated truancy, detention, and suspension from school. They had been linked with a satanic cult that performed rituals and promoted antisocial behavior. After appearing before Bill, the girl, despite her promise in court, did not avoid this group and some time later was found dead. It is conjectured that she was murdered, a victim of this satanic cult.

Drug use is also encouraged in these cults, and violent rituals can be an integral part of membership. As the judge pointed out, the effect of these groups on their members is similar to that of gangs in the inner city. The groups encourage crime, drug use, and violence. They seem consistently linked to the increase in teenage murders throughout the country. Cults seem prevalent in the more affluent, suburban neighborhoods while gangs tend to predominate in the inner city.

Bill and I talked about the impact of abuse on childhood deaths. Viewed from the bench of family court, the incidence of child abuse has increased dramatically. Bill believes that one of the factors contributing to this increased abuse is the growing number children born to teenage mothers. These young women are often single and ill-prepared to handle the responsibilities of child rearing. Consequently, the number of abuse and neglect cases has increased alongside of the rising tide of teen pregnancy. In cases where the child is abused to the point of death, experience has taught Bill that the abuser is often a live-in boyfriend. Bill also points out that although child abuse is reported more frequently than in the past, the systems available to provide follow-up have not received substantial budget increases for more personnel.

Bill laments the lack of responsibility he witnesses in all too many teenage fathers who feel that they can continue to be sexually active without any obligation to use contraception. They act under the false assumption that taking precautions is the girl's responsibility. In some instances, these teenage boys have impregnated several girls and, lacking gainfull employment, are unable to contribute to the child's support. According to Bill, one individual he encountered had impregnated eleven women; for two of these women, it was the second child he had fathered. The real victims here are the children, who must survive without a loving, supportive father.

The judge also hears a lot of cases involving very young children who have been left alone for extended periods. Because inexpensive day care is hard for many parents to find, and because young parents are often immature, their children are left unattended and at great risk for fatal injury—all too often from fires.

Bill believes our present system of dealing with abuse and neglect is inadequate, and that the punishment for these crimes is not harsh enough. He also believes that it is difficult to resolve complex abuse situations. In numerous cases the children want to go home; they are sorry or feel guilty about admitting the abuse. However, Bill believes that such children should not be allowed to return home to their abusive parents until the family has completed counseling. All too often children are returned to the home only to fall victim once again to the vicious cycle of abuse and neglect. Fatal consequences are all too frequent.

To sum up, the problems that Bill feels contribute substantially to the ever-increasing childhood mortality rate are:

1. the growing number of single-parent families in which children do not get the attention and care that they need—this places them at risk for fatal injury and/or behavioral problems that can eventually lead to disaster;

2. the epidemic of illegal drug use: children involved with illegal drugs risk death as users, as dealers, or when committing crimes to support their habit;

3. the inability of present child welfare programs to address the needs of children and their families;

4. the glamorization of sex, violence, and drugs in the media;

5. the disintegration of the traditional nuclear family, which often leads to less supervision and guidance at home—some children give in to peer or gang pressure and run the risk of falling victim to crime and violence as a way of life;

6. the increasing incidence of child abuse;

7. the inability of our present system of law enforcement to deal with drug-related crime and gang violence;

8. the desperation of poverty, which breeds violence and ends in death for many children.

9. We have become a society in which pain and death are normal facts of life to a large portion of our population. We are no longer shocked or horrified by the young people who die in our midst every day. But we should be. We must be!

Some recommendations:

1. We must provide our young children with lots of love and guidance. Help them develop good values and ethics early on. Provide support and education to parents so they can do their best job.

2. Every effort should be made to erradicate the poverty that rests at the core of so many life-threatening problems that are stealing our children from us.

3. Let's make a solid investment in our educational system, because the better educated our children become, the less apt they are to commit crime, become victims of crime, or to engage in dangerous activities such as abusing alcohol and drugs.

4. Our society should stop condoning sexual promiscuity through our failure to combat teenage ignorance about birth control, pregnancy, parenting, and infant care.

5. More stringent guidelines should be drawn to identify suspected child abuse. Parents and adults who abuse, maim, or kill children should be punished to the fullest extent of the law.

6. We need to make sure our children feel good about themselves. We have to teach parents the value of a good home life and the importance of self-esteem.

Throughout all these discussions, it became quite obvious to me that the prevention of childhood death isn't just a problem for parents. While there is much that they can do to safeguard the children in their care, the broader social conditions that lead to life-threatening situations for our youth extend far beyond the ability of any one family to effect a change.

Our system of child welfare is understaffed, underfunded, and overburdened. The number of needy families exceeds the money allocated to help them. All caring adults must be willing to take on more responsibility: we must show a greater interest in our own children, and we have to cooperate with other parents in the community to ensure that programs designed to benefit all children, rich and poor, are available and providing the needed services. Adults throughout this country can no longer afford to ignore the plight of our children.

The issues and problems surrounding child safety and health must become our national priority for the 1990s. I have focused on American children, but the problems plaguing our young people are not unlike those being confronted by parents and adults throughout the world. As a nation we have to work hard to make up for many years of neglect on the child-welfare front. I believe we have made sincere efforts on behalf of children; however, it is equally obvious that a great many problems remain in need of concrete solutions if we are to reduce and eventually eliminate the dangers that claim more and more young lives each year.

As parents we need to be protectors, and as citizens we must become child advocates. Each and every one of us must take a long, hard look at ourselves and the kind of society we want for our children. No problem is insurmountable if we put our minds to it. There are no *easy* solutions but *there are solutions.* The potential for success is there. All we have to do is take the initiative and dedicate ourselves to the task at hand!

Part Three

A Society in Crisis

8

The Underlying Factors

INTRODUCTION

We've discussed at great length the death of children in our society and the reasons for these fatalities. However, up to this point we have been looking at the symptoms rather than the causes of problems that have brought on the high child mortality rate in the United States. Somehow the environment in this country has nurtured and maintained conditions that result in these alarming statistics. But just looking at numbers won't provide much insight if we fail to examine some of the factors that have contributed to the present situation. I don't think it is a simple cause and effect relationship, but rather a combination of complex factors that together have increased the likelihood of these tragedies. In short, the fatalities among our children reflect deep-seated problems in society, which we have all helped to bring about. In the pages that follow, I list some of the more pervasive among them.

1. America has become a "violent society," as our choice of entertainment and amusement can attest. A passing glance at the motion pictures our children watch is ample evidence. In all too many of these films people are not just killed, they are mutilated. I'm not suggesting that all movies are violent and tasteless, but the graphic quality, quantity, duration, and intensity of violence in many films has dramatically increased. And the kids love it! The more violence kids get through entertainment, the more they seem to crave. Violent entertainment is glamorous, profitable, and probably here to stay.

109

But even though some research indicates that such violence might have an impact on levels of violence in the real world as well as increased childhood fears and the incidence of suicide in adolescents, much more research is needed to confirm such a hypothesis (DHHS, 1989). I do believe, however, that our entertainment reflects the desires of a major portion of the population.

We know that parents should monitor what their children view on television and at the movies. The same facts hold true for some popular music, rock videos, and the like. I talk to kids who say "I just like watching and listening; it really doesn't phase me. I know its not real." However, this varies somewhat with the age of the child. Much controversy exists over whether or not this indifference to the media is actually true. I think that what we as a society choose to see and hear may show how our needs and tastes have changed. The nature of the relationship between violent entertainment and social violence is a separate issue and a source of much debate. The fact remains that if our tastes in entertainment show more violence, then does that not reflect a society that has become more violence-prone?

In addition, it is hard to ignore the increases in the numbers of battered wives, abused children, and the increased violence and homicide in our teenagers (Children's Defense Fund, 1989). Violence pervades our lives as well as our entertainment. I'm not an advocate of censorship or restricting First Amendment rights, but at the risk of sounding "preachy," our violent social tendencies are mirrored in the lives of our children. Too many children have fallen victim to it in one form or another. We truly need to address violence in all its forms and increase our sensitivity to it. I believe we must become a "kinder and gentler" nation in every sense of the word.

2. In America, there are a large number of single-parent homes. Some reports indicate that one out of every two or three marriages will end in divorce. Also, for a variety of reasons, some women may choose to remain single parents, while others have been abandoned by their spouse or corresponding parent. Nowadays there are a large number of unplanned teenage pregnancies, and more often than not, these single parents must also work. Even in homes with both parents present, each spouse may need to work to support the family. Therefore, adult supervision and the need for adequate

child care have become recent major social concerns. The available child care doesn't meet this ever-increasing need, and the care that does exist can be either very expensive or substandard.

The need for parents to work has also produced a group of school-age children known as "latchkey" kids—seven million strong—those who must take care of themselves for periods of time before and/or after school. Teenagers may be even more vulnerable to the lack of adult supervision while parents are away from the home working. These adolescents confront a variety of pressures from friends and other peers to engage in unsafe activities and to disregard parental rules.

It is important to remember that there are twenty million working mothers in the United States, over half of whom have children under the age of six (Children's Defense Fund, 1989); our society needs more good, affordable day care and more supervision and guidance for children in every age group.

3. Homelessness has become a critical issue for the 1990s, especially for women and children. By the year 2,000, if current trends continue, millions of American children will have spent at least part of their childhoods without a place to call home (Children's Defense Fund, 1989).

Homelessness carries tremendous implications for children: schooling is disrupted, while health care is either inconsistent or nonexistent. These children are more likely to have chronic illness, elevated levels of lead in their blood, inadequate immunization against childhood diseases, and serious developmental deficiencies and/or psychological conditions (Children's Defense Fund, 1989). Their basic survival needs cannot be met on a regular basis. In many cities, families have to separate to find shelter for all members. The family unit often deteriorates as parents try to survive the hard times and children find themselves placed in foster care or with relatives if the option is available. Because of the stress brought on by the anxiety, frustration, and helplessness of their situation, domestic violence often increases in these families. Desperate parents are often forced to seek housing in abandoned, dangerous buildings when shelters for the homeless cannot make room for them. Existence is a day-to-day affair.

Such dislocation and uncertainty has devastating implications for child care and child rearing: homeless women without money, public assistance, or health insurance tend to lack any prenatal care during a pregnancy. As homelessness and poverty threaten the well-being and survival of more and more Americans, the danger to our children increases and the ranks of the needy and dispossessed swell.

Runaway children compound these problems. Over two thousand children run away every day. A report issued by the Children's Defense Fund states that on any given day in this country, there are one hundred thousand homeless children who need refuge.

Why is the number of homeless women and children on the rise? Alcohol and drug abuse, jobs that pay minimum wage, and overwhelming marital difficulties are the major causes (City Missionary, 1990). Unlike decades past when the neediest among us were society's outcasts, today many rescue missions report that those seeking refuge come from all segments of society. The problems related to homelessness will get worse as public housing opportunities dwindle. Because of inadequate low-cost housing, families are forced to find rental housing. If public assistance funds are inadequate to meet their housing needs, the poor must somehow make up the difference. This has become more and more difficult for increasing numbers of families, who ultimately become homeless.

As a nation, we must do all we can to fund projects that provide support for homeless families. In addition, we need to ensure that the homeless have access to health-care services. Meanwhile, the numbers of low-income housing units should be increased and efforts made to refurbish uninhabitable public housing facilities, the repair of which has been seriously impeded by reductions in funding and past misappropriations of funds.

4. America's health-care delivery system has become ever more conscious of costs. Without a method to pay for care, many families with children do not have access to these needed services. As we have learned, there is inadequate prenatal care for low-income pregnant women and this translates to many low-birth-weight babies. By the year 2,000 the first-year cost for the high-tech care required by all babies born with low birth weight will reach six billion dollars (Children's Defense Fund, 1989).

Poor, uninsured people have very limited use of health-care services and the situation seems to be getting worse. Medicaid reimbursement available for poor parents often falls well below what is considered acceptable payment for health services, so these people may be turned away by medical care providers. Cutbacks in existing though woefully inadequate government funding has significantly limited those remaining free services that are already strained beyond available resources to help less fortunate individuals and families. Even in the situation where one or both parents work, employee insurance programs tend not to cover dependent children as part of the policy. Therefore, these youngsters have no coverage, which has a direct bearing on their access to health-care services. It is often the case, therefore, that a child may be quite ill before emergency medical attention is sought. Even if emergency care is obtained, medications and other treatments may be unavailable or far too expensive.

Additionally, health care for the poor, when it does exist, seems to focus on responding to illness rather than preventive child care. It should also be noted that Medicaid in many states does not cover children beyond the age of six. The "nearly poor" families are many times not poor enough to qualify for Medicaid yet they cannot afford health insurance of any kind.

We need to ensure that all women have access to prenatal care and that all children receive preventive health-care services. Additionally, we have to fight for the expansion of Medicaid and for greater funding to assist maternal child-care programs. All children should have health insurance coverage.

5. Until now, parental child abuse has been ineffectively monitored in many cases. Child protective agencies, whose task it is to respond to complaints involving abuse, are strained to the breaking point. The care or help children and parents receive from child welfare, mental health, and juvenile services may be fragmented and reactive rather than preventive. Counseling for abusers is not consistently available, and preventive services are hard to come by. The availability of adequate foster care may also be problematic. At present, over 250,000 children have alternative living arrangements (Children's Defense Fund, 1989).

There are too many separate but overlapping agencies duplicating inadequate work with abused children, and they are usually bogged down in reams of red tape. There is no centralized national system for keeping track of child-abuse complaints. Once a charge of abuse is rescinded, the record in many cases is erased. Usually, the child must have evidence of extensive physical harm before most states will take action against the abuser(s). Furthermore, the penalties for causing the death of a child due to abuse are not nearly stiff enough (Hawkins, 1986). Over one thousand children died as a result of child abuse in 1987 (Children's Defense Fund, 1989).

Improvements in preventive services and the bolstering of staffs in child-welfare agencies are essential. We must also provide education and counseling on effective parenting to high-risk groups.

6. Alcohol, drugs, and the violence associated with them have gained much national attention; their devastation has rained down upon society for decades with no sign of abating. Individuals die directly and indirectly from the use and abuse of alcohol and drugs. We've already discussed how alcohol contributes to accidents and deaths involving motor vehicles. But these drugs can be lethal all by themselves. A 1989 study of twenty-seven cities found that cocaine—particularly in areas where the crack variety is available—overtook heroin as the single narcotic responsible for the most drug-related deaths.

However, it is important to note that deaths from all *legal* drugs—including prescription amphetamines, barbiturates, and over-the-counter pain killers—are listed on death certificates almost as often as cocaine and heroin combined. An estimated ten to twenty thousand deaths each year are blamed on drug abuse. However, alcohol kills up to ten times more people than all other drugs. Therefore, although much attention is devoted to illegal drugs, we should never underestimate the damage done by legal drugs such as alcohol, prescriptive medications, and over-the-counter remedies.

These days, our teenagers have greater access to alcohol, as evidenced by the fact that 60 percent of high-school seniors consume alcohol on a regular basis (Schulmon, *Buffalo News,* 1990). Illegal drugs are also freely available and more addictive and dangerous than ever. But the huge network of individuals who sell them to our children are protected by the enormous amounts of money generated by the sale of these drugs. Drugs are big business, but our government has been slow and ineffective in its response to the threat. Many children are in violent neighborhoods where the menace of drugs is everywhere and parents find themselves powerless to protect the safety and well-being of their own offspring. These neighborhoods are also plagued by gang-related violence that places a major strain on law enforcement in many urban areas. These gang activities are consistently linked to illegal drugs.

The media and highly visible celebraties, such as rock stars and professional athletes, often are responsible for glamorizing drugs and alcohol. Our children are impressed by the slick beer commercials and by powerful role models whose actual or reported drug use encourages large numbers of teens to experiment with drugs and alcohol. As discussed previously, alcohol plays a part in many teenage deaths involving motor vehicles. In fact, in over half the accidents involving teens, the driver (also a teen) was intoxicated.

Besides being the culprit in teenage drinking and driving accidents, alcohol and other drugs also influence teen sexual behaviors. A survey conducted on college-age students reported that alcohol and other drugs influenced the students' decision in 37 percent of the cases to engage in sexual activity when they were otherwise unsure of what they wanted; 34 percent reported at least once that intoxication was used as an excuse for sexual activity; and 18 percent reported using coercion or aggression while under the influence to engage in sexual activity (*CV*, 1990).

7. We need to do more research on diseases for which there are no known cures, such as "crib death" (SIDS) among infants and AIDS throughout the population. AIDS was ignored for too long in the high-risk populations and allowed to spread too far before any preventive action was taken. The early lack of knowledge regarding the monitoring of this disease in blood products resulted in the infection of people who had merely received transfusions. The sharing of needles by drug addicts also became a mechanism for spreading the disease. Women who slept with these intravenous drug users became infected and passed this disease on to their unborn children. As a result, the disease spread to the heterosexual population.

Much misconception and lack of knowledge surrounds the health problem posed by AIDS. Money earmarked for research and treatment is now more available. However, in the years since its first detection, the number of AIDS cases has increased dramatically. AIDS will take an increasing toll on families and children in the next decade. The Centers for Disease Control projects ten thousand cases of childhood AIDS by 1991 (Children's Defense

Fund, 1989), yet we still have very limited research and care facilities dedicated to the victims of this disease.

It also now appears that the AIDS epidemic may spread to our teen population. Sharp increases in the number of teens testing positive has caused a growing concern among youth-care workers that adolescents are the next "hot spot" in this epidemic. High-risk behaviors (promiscuity) plus the lack of practical prevention place this group at a substantially increased risk (*AIDS Newsletters of WNY,* 1990). Results of testing in subgroups demonstrate its prevalence in older teens. About one to two individuals out of every one thousand military recruits and one out of every five hundred college students tested in a recent national study (the majority were eighteen to twenty-four years old) tested positive for the virus (*AIDS Newsletters of WNY,* 1990). We need a national plan to combat this lethal disease.

8. We have to attack racial, sexual, and ethnic injustice and discrimination of all types. As a society we have thrived on the variety and differences in the ethnic and racial groups that make up our country. It has been a historical formula for our national success. If we are to survive and prosper as a nation, then every citizen must have an equal opportunity to succeed.

We still have not achieved equality. In fact, incidents of discrimination are on the rise. There is documentation to show that the occurrence of racial intolerance and violence is building among our young people, especially on college campuses. According to a recent college magazine, reports of campus harassment due to some sort of discrimination have increased as much as 400 percent since 1985. African-Americans drop out of all-white schools at a rate five times higher than whites at the same school. The Anti-Defamation League reports a six-fold increase in anti-Semitic episodes on campuses between 1985 and 1988 (Shenk, 1990). This reflects a failure on the part of all adults of all races, cultures, and political persuasions to deal with these prejudices and to make our country a healthy, cohesive nation. If we impose economic sanctions on South Africa for practicing white supremacy, we need also to deal with this problem here in our own backyard.

Every American must have the same chance to flourish, but statistics demonstrate that citizens of nonwhite ethnic groups do not have the same choices or chances from birth to adulthood as those of the majority white groups. Our children's welfare is the best measure of quality and although Caucasian children die unnecessarily, our African-American children are at greater risk of death at almost any age. Leaders representing all races, cultures, and ethnic groups must fight for all children and foster tolerance and understanding in all our future citizens.

> So the machine has melted, the phone has stretched to where it is useless. This is how intense the heat is. Liberals, who largely control the administration, faculty, and students' rights groups of leading academic institutions, have, with virtually no intensive intellectual debate, inculcated schools with their answers to the problem of bigotry. Conservatives, with a long history of insensitivity to minority concerns, have been all but shut out of the debate, and now want back in. Their intensive pursuit of the true nature of bigotry and the proper response to it—working to assess the "real needs" of campuses rather than simply bowing to pressure—deserves to be embraced by all concerned parties, and probably would have been by now but for two small items: (a) Reagan, their fearless leader, was clearly insensitive to ethnic/feminist concerns; and (b) some of the more coherent conservative pundits still show a blatant apathy to the problems of bigotry in this country. This has been sufficient ammunition for liberals who are continually looking for an excuse to keep conservatives out of the dialogue. So now we have clashes rather than debates: on how much one can say, on how much one should have to hear. Two negatives: one side wants to crack down on expression, the other on awareness. The machine has melted, and it's going to take some consensus to build a new one. Intellectual provincialism will have to end before young hate ever will (Shenk, 1990, p. 39).

9. Teenage pregnancy has reached epidemic proportions. Each day, approximately two to three thousand teens get pregnant; and during the same period over twelve hundred give birth. Of these, over six hundred teens have inadequate prenatal care (Children's Defense Fund, 1990). This has tremendous implications for both health care and infant mortality. Teen pregnancy is not a new phenomena.

However, its implications for child welfare in this day and age cannot be ignored. Many teenage mothers do not finish high school, which seriously impedes their ability to support themselves and their children. Additionally, the number of teens who do not marry has quadrupled since 1960 (Children's Defense Fund, 1989). So although the teen pregnancy rate has declined, the number of out-of-wedlock children has substantially increased. Adolescent boys are, for the most part, financially incapable of supporting the children they father. These problems have tremendous economic ramifications for our society as we approach the next century.

We must increase access to family planning and expand services to teen parents. We have to reach those with a high risk of early parenthood through programs specifically geared to them. Programs need to be developed for adolescent boys so that they are integrated into pregnancy-prevention strategies. Parents should ensure that their sexually active children have access to birth control information and strategies. We must instill in young men accountability for the fathering of unwanted children. An all-out attack must be waged on any double standard that allows men to have sex without consequence. In addition, young women must be persuaded to practice contraception if they are sexually active.

A young fifteen-year-old girl said to me that she felt the only productive thing she would ever do in her life would be to have a child. This was her way of making a contribution to and leaving her mark on society. It made me very sad that she thought this was the best choice she could make at such a young age. What made her think it was her only alternative? I seriously doubted that this bright, energetic child had no other creative outlet, yet it's easy to see why she would feel this way. We idealize single motherhood in the media (look at all the stars who choose to be single parents), and we fail to educate kids about the tremendous responsibilities that go along with parenting and raising a child.

I talked with some young men (eighteen- to nineteen-year-olds) about teenage pregnancy. I found that only a few of them use a condom, and their rationale for using one was to prevent exposure to sexually transmitted diseases rather than to prevent pregnancy. I certainly don't mean to imply that this is reflective of all young men; however, I do believe that the fact that only one out of the five was using a condom and all were sexually active warrants attention. I asked them whether they would ask a girl with whom they were going to have sexual relations if she used any contraceptive method. All said they probably would not. I asked what they would do if the girl became pregnant. All said, they would first have to be convinced it was their child, and if paternity was established, all said they would try to find a "way out." None said they would marry the girl, or willingly support the child. One young man expressed resentment over the fact that the girl had the right to decide to go ahead with the pregnancy even if the father objected. Food for thought.

I have also talked with teenage girls and found that a good number did not use any form of contraception. This is evident in the literature since less than one-third are reported to use any type of birth control method even when sexually active (Children's Defense Fund, 1989). Being a woman, I have often felt that pregnancy was ultimately the woman's choice. It interested me that these young people felt little responsibility for the consequences of their sexual activity. Duly impressed, I immediately talked with my own son; I suppose I assumed that my values were his. I have always emphasized "safe sex" from the perspective of sexually transmitted diseases. I have also tried to impress upon my children the necessity of birth control and accountability for one's decisions. However, I have probably done more of the latter with my daughter. I have since initiated steps to remedy the situation.

Children of both sexes need to be educated to the fact that teenage pregnancy results in a great number of high-risk infants. The death toll among these infants could be reduced substantially if we addressed the practices and responsibility of sexually active teenagers.

In conclusion, I did ask one of the boys what he would do if a girl with whom he had had casual sex became pregnant, decided to have the child, and sued him for support. His answer may have been fictitious: "I'd kill her." Maybe this young man's attitude is not reflective of most teenage men. However, it is hard to ignore that although the number of teen pregnancies has been substantially reduced since the 1960s, only 15 percent of those babies were born out of wedlock. Today, 60 percent of the babies born to teenage mothers are born outside of marriage (Children's Defense Fund, 1989). Therefore, more and more of these pregnant teens become dependent on a system that is not adequate to cope with the current situation, and many of their children are born only to become infant mortality statistics.

10. Americans must deal with a crisis in education. Good quality schools should be available for all children; every effort must be made to reverse the deterioration of many of our schools. We must equip our teachers and educational leaders with the resources they need to provide the best possible education to all children. Every child should have the opportunity to learn a skill or obtain an education that will allow them to support themselves and their future families.

Our schools have suffered immeasurably from reduced funding and neglect. We are trying to be competitive with other nations even to the extent of lengthening the school year. I'm not an expert, but I do believe that quality is more important than the quantity of time spent in school. Have we really invested in quality? Education has been one of the first areas cut when a budget crunch occurs, not just at the federal but at the state and local levels, too. How many valuable services that schools provide have been cut? With proper support and funding can schools safeguard our children's health and safety when they are away from home?

My teacher friends have told me that they feel a great deal of pressure to help "at risk" or endangered kids. They work overtime to do everything possible because for many of these children they are the adults with whom the kids have the most contact. However, there is a limit to the teachers' time and the resources available to them. Poor, disadvantaged youth are especially prone to fall behind their more affluent peers. Poverty can often be related to poor skills, higher school drop-out rates, and missed opportunities for college. Poor children are more likely to attend schools that are struggling to make ends meet with inadequate resources (Children's Defense Fund, 1989). Perhaps, the only way to really eliminate poverty is to invest in our educational system.

Significant decreases in financial aid, when combined with skyrocketing college tuitions, have successfully denied many young people access to college. The Children's Defense Fund recommends increasing the number of needy children who have access to Chapter 1 programs (remedial programs for poor children). The growing number of non-English and handicapped children must have access to expanded federally funded programs as outlined in the Education for All Handicapped Children Act and the Bilingual Education Act. As a middle-class parent, I feel the federal government needs to provide further subsidy for college costs; I've been barely able to keep up with these tuition costs because loans available to students are not indexed to the costs of college tuition. Parents must make up the difference. Even a moderately successful professional has a difficult time coming up with the necessary additional funds. Disadvantaged youths are not able to make up this difference. They need support services like Head Start and Upward Bound to help ready them for their secondary and postsecondary education. They need help with college expenses!

11. Lack of (or decreases in) government funding and changes in the distribution of these funds for social programs have significantly cut back many available services to the needy. This has caused decreases not only in the quantity but the quality of services, which to the needy are already fragmented and inadequate. An emphasis on "volunteerism" has now become a major thrust for making up the deficits in many social programs as well as child-welfare-related services.

   Is volunteerism a real solution? While it certainly may not be the answer to all our problems, there is no doubt that we have to do more for our children with a lot less money. Are the agencies that do exist really responsive to the needs of all children or have they become so complex and administratively top-heavy that they may fail the mission for which they exist? To whom are they accountable?

   When a teenage acquaintance was badly burned, I was amazed how little could be done to help him. He was either too young for help from some services or too old for help from other organizations. He fell into the cracks. We see this happening with far too many children.

   Perhaps we have to really look at the resources various child-welfare agencies have and who they really serve. How can we make them more effectively meet the needs of children in this country (Kimmick, 1985)?

12. Politically children have no power. They have few sponsors or "lobbyists" when it comes to politics, and they don't vote. Many times laws or programs that benefit children are tied to controversial political issues like abortion. Restrictions on abortion are seen by some politicians as pro-child measures. While I won't argue one way or another on this issue, the controversy can divert atten-

tion away from other bills and programs that directly benefit children.

The individual states enact many laws and administer programs that protect children. They vary from state to state and therefore efforts to reform or change them can be complex. Children's programs that are truly successful are characterized by dedicated staffs, comprehensive services, and committed parents. All these ingredients are hard to find in every community and therefore some services just can't do the best job. The situation needs to be altered.

We need to be aware of how our elected representatives vote with regard to child-welfare issues. The Children's Defense Fund, an advocacy group for kids, has two persons now assigned to its government-affairs section. KIDSPAC, a lobbying group for children, has hired a full-time employee. However, we all need to be "lobbyists" for children's issues (Whitman et al., 1988).

13. Poverty is a major factor having an impact on the general welfare of children. Of all the major industrialized countries, our poverty rate in the United States is two to three times higher (Children's Defense Fund, 1989). Of all the problems we have discussed, poverty is most pervasive and it overlaps many of the other factors we've addressed. The truth is, our poorest children are more at risk of death!

I was recently reading a current edition of *National Geographic* (May 1990), in which one of the articles addressed growing up in East Harlem (New York City). It is a written and pictorial essay of poverty within the boundaries of one of this country's largest cities. East Harlem is primarily African-American and Hispanic, among whom those without jobs account for one in seven, while one in three gets some form of public assistance. It is a crime-ridden area characterized by an increasing use of drugs, a high incidence of AIDS, and escalating high-school dropout rates (VanDyk, 1990). The article depicts life in the "barrio," from the man selling drugs openly on the corner to a picture of the child born addicted to cocaine screaming in the foreground of a photograph, while his uncle sells cocaine over the phone in the background. Drugs, crime, and horror come home to haunt us in these pages. Change may be coming slowly to this area, due in part to the multiple generations of people on welfare, but there is still hope. Educators, religious leaders, economic incentives, and many dedicated people are working hard to promote change.

This neighborhood, like many poverty-stricken neighborhoods across the country, needs public support and funding to reverse the horror of poverty. It is easy to see why the children of poverty are so vulnerable. Until we deal with the circumstances surrounding poverty, we will be unable to save a large portion of our children who are at risk. They have too many obstacles to overcome. Poverty breeds the kind of situations within society that contribute to the death of many children each year. According to the Children's Defense Fund (1989), it is estimated that with an expenditure of fifty-two billion dollars we could eliminate poverty for all people in America. That sounds like a lot of money to be sure, until we consider that it's no more than the base price for a new Stealth B-2 Bomber. Our national priorities should change. We need to invest that money in the future of our children.

I have tried to touch on some of the social problems that combine to create an environment that ultimately contributes to devastation and death among America's children. The components of this environment become more vivid when we think about how our children die. We can prevent many of their deaths by focusing on the causes and then determining strategies to help not only our own children but the youth of America as well to survive and grow to productive adulthood.

Part Four

Evaluating the
Role of Government

9

Current Status of Government and Voluntary Agency Programs for Children

Wanda Therolf, Attorney at Law

Previous chapters have detailed the many ways in which the lives of our children are threatened. We should all be very concerned about this dangerous trend in our society. The loss of our children means the loss of our future. Over the years and to varying degrees federal, state, and local governments have developed and instituted a wide array of programs to help our nation's youth. Legislation was enacted to provide for basic protection of young and old alike. For example, the Food and Drug Administration (FDA) has attempted to regulate the purity and safety of ingredients found in food products and medications so that minimum standards are maintained. The Consumer Product Safety Commission (CPSC) continues to struggle with dwindling resources but has managed to persevere in its aggressive attitude toward protecting children from dangerous toys.

According to the CPSC, over 100,000 children under the age of fifteen were treated for toy-related injuries in hospital emergency rooms in 1987. Thirty-seven reported deaths from January 1987 to September 1988 were directly linked to toy-related accidents. Unfortunately, the CPSC has also experienced funding cuts that have resulted in the reduction of its nationwide network of area offices from fourteen to three. Product liability laws have been passed to try to fill in the gap, but this legislation is triggered only when a serious injury or death occurs.

I will discuss, albeit briefly, the effect that budget cuts enacted by

President Reagan in the early 1980s have had on the lives of our children. A large percentage of the young people who die are children of poor and lower-middle-class families; the impact of events on their parents both directly and indirectly affects the well-being of these children.

During the 1960s and 1970s, government was in a position to establish programs that would provide a wide variety of assistance to the poor and disadvantaged and add to existing programs as new needs were identified. Programs designed to deal with nutrition, housing, health care, safety, education, and employment were created and funded by the federal government. Areas such as special education, day care, recreation, and job training were all part of the federal plan to help the needy. During this time of broad-based public assistance, it was discovered that an increasingly large number of children were living in poverty and that a significant portion of them were from single-parent families, which were usually headed by the mother. By 1981 more than 20 percent of all children in the United States lived in poverty and 47 percent of these youngsters were African-American.

In 1981 President Ronald Reagan signed into law the Omnibus Budget Reconciliation Act, which sounded the death knell for most if not all of the programs that had previously been enacted by the federal government. This act transferred much of the responsibility for funding and policy setting for these programs away from the federal government and into the hands of state and local governments as well as the private sector. The reduced federal role in the area of children's services sparked a downward spiral of change in the delivery of those services and in the opportunity for children to receive them.

In 1985 and 1986 the federal budget included even more severe cuts in children's programs: aid to special education, community-service block grants, summer youth employment, runaway and homeless youth, food stamps, child nutrition, aid to families with dependent children (AFDC), and Medicaid experienced significantly reduced levels of funding. Severe restraints were also placed on juvenile-justice, delinquency-prevention, and legal-services programs as well as Head Start, job-training partnerships, job corp, and many other programs that were specifically designed for or included the enhancement of children's lives.

Years of accumulated evidence testify to the fact that children continue to suffer from the ravages of poverty; this is particularly true of minority children and those who live in single-parent environments with a female head of the household. Everyone knows that with the breakup of a marriage or a family setting, the mother usually shoulders the burden of providing for the children. Without financial assistance from the father the income and overall economic status of the mother and her children take a dramatic turn for the worse. This financial downturn usually forces the mother/head of household to seek assistance from federal or state agencies in order to provide the basic necessities of daily life for her children: food, shelter, and clothing.

In order to understand the effect of the shift in funding from the federal government to the state and local authorities, it is helpful to understand how the funding actually works. The federal government establishes a specific program and arranges for funding by allotting a portion of the federal budget to that program. The standards that must be met to qualify for the program are established and a bureaucracy is formed to deal with the internal functioning of the program as well as the external or distribution portion of the program. Staff must be found and paid and records must be kept so that an accounting of the funds distributed can be reconciled with the funds received. As new areas of need are identified, new programs are developed or older programs are adapted to meet these needs. Over time the federal government had established numerous programs and had invested many millions of dollars each year to maintain them.

Specific rules were established with regard to spending the programs' funds. Criteria or standards of need were identified and formalized by legislation. Cutoffs were determined based on annual family income or the age of the children to be served.

As the federal government shifted more and more of the burden of supporting these programs onto state and local authorities, the resources became increasingly limited. State and local governments have attempted to deal with the problem of reduced funding by trying to obtain the money from their own general funds and by moving funds from other social services. This involves a shifting of costs to another program such as AFDC (e.g., child-care provisions) and Medicaid (e.g., homemaker services). However, day-care programs have suffered greatly; to shore up the gaps, the states have turned to local providers who offer a "service for a fee," making it almost impossible for the working poor to afford quality affordable care. For example, a woman must decide if she wants to work and pay the fee for child-care services (for some this is not an option because they simply can't afford the fee), work and give their children a key to let themselves in (latchkey children form a large part of the poor population), or stay home with her children and live on Welfare. (This option is also difficult to choose since the qualifying standard is constantly being raised;

more and more of the poor are not able to qualify for Welfare benefits, and even if they did qualify, they might not meet the eligibility requirements for other programs that are necessary for survival.)

For those families who do qualify for Medicaid health benefits, there are still problems. Reduced funding resulted in staff cuts at the clinics, which have, in turn, resulted in less staff available for care, longer waiting times, less hours allotted for appointments, and fewer services being offered. Clients were forced to come up with a copayment and general eligibility requirements were changed, all of which made Medicaid less accessible to poor families.

State and local support has attempted to replace some of this lost funding, but they have been unable for the most part to keep up with each new round of federal budget cuts. Some states were not in a position to pick up the extra costs, while other states took advantage of federal cutbacks to reduce general assistance and overall costs. The Reagan administration insisted that the private sector (nonprofit agencies) could and would help. Unfortunately, it was not easy for them to do.

These agencies are now overburdened on the one hand by the increasing numbers of people who need their help, and on the other as a result of lost funding due to cutbacks in service contracts. To some extent, these private agencies were able to compensate for various losses by increasing their service fees and charges. This, however, makes it more difficult to provide assistance to the nonpaying persons who have also lost their public benefits and who find themselves more than ever in need of help. In order to cope with these cutbacks, families have had to settle for lower-quality care or no care at all. This also makes it very difficult to improve the level of service to families with young children who desperately need medical care and nutrition to ensure their proper growth and development.

Everyone has heard of Third World countries and their high death rates and low standards of living. The United States has its own Third World country within its borders. Our poor, including the children, make up this "country" and its population is growing steadily.

Often families turn to what are referred to as last-resort programs. These service providers offer supplementary food for women, infants, and children (WIC), general assistance, or outpatient hospital care. Congress has attempted to address the growing demands on social services by creating the House Select Committee on Children, Youth, and Families. In 1981 the median income of mother-only families was $8,653, which was 34 percent of that earned by husband-wife families during the same period. Twenty percent of all children live in poverty, with African-American children being about three times more likely to be poor than white children.

Children and their families need supportive services, especially aid to families with dependent children (AFDC), Medicaid, and food stamps. The states spend about half their funds from social-service grants on child-welfare services, which have experienced significant reductions in funding —anywhere from 20 to 64 percent, once an adjustment for inflation has been made. These programs include foster care, adoption, protective services such as preventing child-abuse and neglect, child-care programs (eliminated in 1986), Head Start (this program has been receiving increased federal funding, the only program which can make that claim), and Judicial Justice and Delinquency Prevention, which has benefited from the state justice bill but remains at about 6 percent below costs.

The Community Services Administration is now incorporated into the Department of Health and Human Services; this agency helped to provide funds for health, nutrition, housing, and employment services for low-income families. The focus of these various programs was to benefit poor families with children, but they fell victim to the budget-cutting axe, losing about 61 percent of their funding in the early 1980s, and despite some gains in the mid 1980s, they have remained consistently below the necessary levels of funding. This has affected services for the prevention of lead-based paint poisoning, genetics and hemophilia projects, and disabled children's programs, although maternal and infant care remain a high priority. In order to concentrate on caring for mothers and their children, other areas that also required funding but were not considered to be as important saw even more substantial cuts in funding since monies ordinarily used for their programs were funneled into these core programs.

Programs that attempted to address the needs of children in the area of preventive health services, such as alcohol and drug abuse, mental health, health education, risk reduction, smoking and substance abuse in secondary schools, hypertension, fluoridation, urban rat control, and emergency medical services, were cut back drastically or eliminated altogether. The comprehensive health services, which were used to support such local health department programs as childhood immunization and adolescent family life programs, with a core offering of prenatal and pediatric services, have seen an increase in some funding, but the money is allocated on a competitive basis to public or nonprofit organizations.

The food-stamp program is one of several nutritional programs created to benefit children and their families. About eleven million people rely on food coupons for support. The food-stamp rolls expanded as the numbers of poor and unemployed people began to increase. In order to meet the demand for assistance, eligibility requirements were tightened, thereby reducing the number of people who could qualify for benefits. Although putting in place new restrictions did help to curb the pressure for funds to support the program, it did not affect the number of people who needed help; it merely decreased the number of persons who actually received food stamps. With the reduced availability of food stamps, school-based food programs were about the only remaining way to guarantee that children ate well at least once during the day. On an average day, over 23.6 million children received lunch at minimal or no cost to the families. This funding was cut by the Reconciliation Act because the Reagan administration felt that too many children whose families were not actually poor were getting free meals. However, 80 percent of low-income children were provided with lunch from this funding and 95 percent received a good breakfast.

The Women, Infants, and Children Program, or WIC, is a supplemental food program of last resort, providing nutritional supplements to 2.4 million people. But funding has not kept pace with the demands on the program: WIC has been forced to drop its cutoff age from four years to one year in order to maintain a smaller deficit in funding. Each year the program barely keeps pace with the increased demand for benefits and the rate of inflation.

The fate of poor children hangs on the intricacies of the Aid to Families with Dependent Children (AFDC) program, which provides much-needed income. Almost all AFDC assistance goes to female heads of households. More than 7 million children in 3.6 million families receive this aid, and for most of these families their very existence depends on the benefits they receive. It's frightening that a few changes in the laws can have such a far-reaching effect on our children's lives and their futures. With each change that the Reconciliation Act made in the eligibility requirements, AFDC was compelled to cut back, further reducing or eliminating benefits. One such change was that pregnant women received no benefits before the sixth month of pregnancy. As we have learned in previous chapters, adequate nutrition during the early stages of pregnancy is vital to assure proper growth and development of the fetus. When poor nutrition among expectant mothers is coupled with the lack of good medical care during infancy the risks escalate that infant and child death will be the inevitable result.

State and local government support was expected to pick up the slack created by massive federal budget cuts. For the most part the support has been forthcoming but a great deal of economic stress on communities has been created as well. Three areas have been well supported by state and local governments: maternal and child health; preventive health service; and alcohol, drug abuse, and mental health. Programs in these areas were given priority for funding. Some states were able to compensate for each dollar of federal aid that was cut, although other states were frequently not able to match amounts, nor were they able to compensate for the effects of inflation. Often the states only concentrated on portions of various programs while ignoring the rest. Though the most essential services were maintained on the state level, there was a price to be paid. Many states managed to fund one program by reducing their commitment to others. Some states, such as New York, enacted the Child Welfare Reform Act, which contained provisions for cost sharing to encourage local (county and city) development of prenatal and supportive services.

This replacement technique is one way for state governments to compensate for losses in one specific area by using funds from other sources. If a state fails to spend (or does not plan to spend) all the money allocated to one or more specific programs, it may transfer a limited amount of these funds to another program where additional allocations are needed. States use this shifting of funds to maximize the level of federal support for the services provided. However, state and local governments are now providing the majority of funds to support state child-welfare services and their respective contributions to health programs appear to be on the increase.

Certain programs appear to be given higher priority for funding. Social services is one such area of public assistance: even when budget constraints force cutbacks, the funding reductions are focused on those categories considered to be least essential, such as day care, since it is not considered a crisis service. Maternal and child health services as well as crippled children's services fared better in the competition for public funds than did public awareness programs about the dangers of lead-based poisoning, support for SIDS research, and adolescent pregnancy programs. With a great deal of advocacy work and public pleading, many needed public assistance services have managed to survive, but their ability to provide consistent levels of support for those who need it most is often undermined by the effects of inflation. The money allocated just doesn't go far enough.

The federal Reconciliation Act mandated changes in the Medicaid program, which gave the states more discretion over services offered and payment mechanisms. In other words, the states had more control over who was offered what services and how much was to be charged for the services by way of a copayment. In addition, the federal government reduced its funding for various educational services to the poor. This forced similar reductions on the state and local levels, which means that only the most necessary services are provided for first, with little or no monies left to be distributed to any of the other programs. Shifts in funding Medicaid have potentially worsened the health-care situation for families by reducing optional services and increasing copayment requirements.

Understandably, when budget crunches occur critical needs are often met before prevention needs can be addressed. But what our politicians fail to grasp is that without programs in place to promote good nutrition and health care, there will always be crises of one kind or another. Relying on stop-gap measures will not do.

In some instances, the states shift some portion of the expense for a specific program onto the county but do not provide matching funds to cover the costs. On other occasions, the states give local governments reduced funds in a lump sum and then allow the county or city governments various degrees of discretion in distributing the cutback. Other state strategies include not reimbursing local governments for the full cost of a program, or transferring funds to specific grants and forcing the counties or cities to match the funds.

As reductions take place in government programs, it has been expected that nonprofit, voluntary, or charity groups would fill in the gap. However, these organizations have also been directly affected by budget cuts. Since a portion of their income is derived from government grants, as these grants decrease, the operating budgets of such groups decline. At all levels of public assistance, nonprofit agencies see their sources of funding drying up while the need for their services continues to grow.

Most nonproft agencies for children received some form of funding from one or more levels of government, with the average agency receiving about 40 percent of its budget requirement. To augment their support, these agencies had to turn to other methods of funding: fees, dues, service charges, and contributions. This of course created problems since the government-funded programs are geared to the poor, the very people who most require the services. A serious question presented itself: Who shall receive the service, those who cannot pay but who are most in need of the services or those who can pay?

Nonprofit agencies provide services that complement the efforts of public service providers. Thus they enjoy a degree of autonomy that permits them to focus on sometimes very specialized needs in the community. But these agencies are often forced to change their focus because of a shift to reliance on the other sources of funding. There has been a shift away from social and educational services toward health and recreation needs; the former are the most income-dependent services dealing with family stress from unemployment, single parenthood, and other factors that lead to low income. As money continues to be cut from publically funded programs, poor and needy children will suffer. The future of children's services is uncertain, but the trend seems to tell a story of irreversible decline.

Responsibility for aiding the neediest children in society has been passed down from federal to state to local government, to nonprofit service providers, and finally to service recipients (the public). Coping strategies have decreased as did discretionary resources for individuals who were responsible for making choices about how to deal with the reduction of services that were presently available. Some families defer routine care or settle for lower-quality care, while others turn to last-resort programs such as special supplemental food programs for women, infants, and children; general assistance programs; or hospital outpatient departments. Because routine care is deferred and forcing families to utilize services less suited to their needs, children are more often facing crisis situations that require outside help immediately. Thus, hospital outpatient departments and emergency rooms are overcrowded with people seeking emergency care and non-emergency health care. Locally funded general assistance or general relief programs for income support are inundated with urgent requests for aid, while WIC programs and local soup kitchens are straining to meet the needs of the poor and the homeless. It is very difficult to determine accurately the number of families that are forced to find help. Emergency-room utilization figures often don't distinguish between actual emergencies and minor problems that could have been routinely treated at a clinic, and soup kitchens don't ask their patrons if they have lost their food stamps or AFDC benefits. Requests for aid not covered by federal funds are frequently shifted to other programs, which offer services that might be less helpful to the needy or are provided at a much higher cost per person.

Local neighborhood clinics, a primary source of health care for poor families and their children, have been negatively affected by the reduction in maternal and child health-care funds and by restrictions in Medicaid coverage, which had included prescriptions, laboratory work, and reimbursement for individual physicians. The clinics must now curtail services or refer nonpaying clients to other providers, such as the outpatient departments of local hospitals.

Public and nonprofit hospitals are also suffering from this downward spiral. Medicaid constraints have caused them to reduce their overall services to poor families. Some hospitals are limiting the number of patients they will admit, which in effect restricts care to a small portion of those who cannot pay or those without third-party coverage.

Poor families, including the children, are affected twice by all these reductions. Proper health care has become significantly less available to them and they are finding it increasingly more difficult to feed and clothe their children. It is very hard to separate the effects of cutbacks in human services during the Reagan administration, as numerous as they were, from the impact of the recession or from the fiscal difficulties of individual states. All have worked together to create the almost impossible situation that now exists for our nation's poor. The stress level is evidenced by the growing number of reports of child abuse and neglect, the increased use of hospital emergency rooms, and the many reported cases of malnutrition.

There have been some very recent national initiatives with regard to maternal and child health that may have implications for social service efforts to stem the tide of childhood death. According to the Children's Defense Fund, recent strides have been made to improve the nation's public system of paying for and delivering medical care.

1. Congress has enacted laws that will substantially increase the number of pregnant women and those with babies who will be eligible to receive Medicaid coverage as of July 1990. Congress has also given states the option of extending Medicaid to all children younger than age eight in families with incomes less than the federal poverty level. There will also be Medicaid coverage available to families who are making the transition from welfare to work for a period of one year after their employment begins.

2. Washington has appropriated sufficient funds to the federal immunization program to purchase the vaccine needed to immunize fully all our infants, toddlers, and preschoolers.

3. Sufficient funds have been added to federal community and migrant centers to permit the establishment of maternal and infant health care services at about half of these centers.

This is a summary of some recent steps that have been taken; however, more needs to be done. According to the Children's Defense Fund, we should finish the Medicaid expansion, increase funding for public health programs, and revitalize the National Health Service Corps. This corps provides scholarship and loan repayment to health professionals who will agree to exchange work in underserved geographic areas where health care is not adequate. In addition, states should move to bolster WIC programs.

There must be more support for child-care programs, child safety, and services for high-risk youths and adolescents. All levels of government must move to correct the obvious deficiencies that have led to alarmingly high rates of childhood death in these groups.

Part Five

The Challenge and Responsibility of Safeguarding Our Children

10

Learn about Your Child's Growth and Development

INTRODUCTION

If we parents and concerned adults are to develop solutions to the life-threatening conditions that claim all too many precious young lives, we must come to understand how our own children grow and develop. It is particularly vital that expectant mothers are educated regarding child growth and development. Adults who are well versed in these stages of a child's physical and emotional maturity will be better prepared to spot changes that seem abnormal or uncharacteristic. In other words, knowledge of how children develop could help us pinpoint danger signs before a life-threatening situation occurs. Though I can only sketch information here, many fine sources are available at the public library or your local bookstore. What is important is that parents take the time to read about the psychological and physiological processes that their children experience when growing up. If necessary, a professional should be consulted.

Just spending time with a youngster can help parents to know and understand their child's behavior and recognize when something *just doesn't seem right*. It is always better to be cautious. Those who ignore a small problem because they think it's silly may be overlooking the initial stage of something far more serious. Many times friends in the nursing profession have told me that during a routine checkup a mother will tell them something about her child's health or behavior that eventually leads to a quite unexpected discovery. For example, a mother may ask why her baby boy has a rash when he eats certain types of food or formula. Such information may not be evident during the exam, because the symptoms may not be present. (Remember, physicians and other health-care providers are not in a position to observe the child regularly as the parent is.) The mother should not be reluctant to ask the doctor or nurse for advice. In most instances, her curiosity or concern helps the health-care provider reevaluate the child's situation and possibly uncover a condition before it has a chance to cause a serious health problem.

Parents, always be on the alert; observe and listen to your children. Be familiar with what is considered normal growth, development, and behavior for infants or for the particular age group of your child(ren). Never be reluctant to ask questions about their health and welfare.

GROWTH AND DEVELOPMENT: AN OVERVIEW

Theories of child development abound: some hold that what a child becomes is largely a matter of biology or genetics, while others propose that the child is a product of both his biology and the environment in which he is reared. Still other theories build on the interaction of genetics and maturation to detail sequential types of developmental tasks for the various stages of growth throughout childhood. Probably the best known theories about the stages of growth are those outlined by Sigmund Freud. However, Eric Erickson and Jean Piaget are also leading theorists in the psychosocial growth and development of children. Their theories describe experiences at various stages of growth and how skills that develop in each are built on preceding stages. Additionally, there are theories of how children learn to interpret the environment.

No matter what theory of development is utilized, it has been established that there are particular kinds of skills and developmental tasks that the growing child should acquire or be capable of at specific periods in life. Children who deviate substantially from these norms may indeed be in need of professional assistance. If parents are to be fully equipped in the battle to safeguard their children, they must have an awareness of these developmental milestones so that potential problems can be spotted early.

Certain principles are universally accepted, the first being that *development progresses from head to foot*. This is demonstrated by the fact that the baby's head is much larger in proportion to its body size at birth. The trunk is also much larger in relation to body size in the infant than in the adult, whereas the legs of an adult are proportionately longer than those of the infant. From birth to adulthood, the rate of growth is greatest in the lower body. Therefore, physical growth follows this head-to-toe pattern.

The development of the baby's motor skills—the ability to move—also follows this pattern. A baby first learns to move its head, then it sits up, crawls, creeps, and eventually walks alone.

The second principle is that *development progresses from a central axis right down the center of the body out to the end of the extremities.* In other words, large-muscle control (e.g., shoulders and hips) is acquired before the small-muscle control (e.g., arms, legs, feet, and hands). This control proceeds down the extremities. For instance, infants can wave their arms and grasp objects with the whole hand before using two fingers in a pincer-type movement to grasp an object. A child can learn to walk long before mastering the ability to dial a telephone.

Third is the principle that *a child learns from general to specific.* New infants will cry whenever they are uncomfortable, whereas older children cry in response to specific noxious stimuli.

Growth and development of particular body systems and body parts occur at different rates and at different times during childhood. This is the fourth principle to remember. Growth does not occur at a steady pace, nor do all body parts develop simultaneously. For instance, an adolescent girl develops mature breasts during the process of puberty, while muscles and nerves are developing from the very earliest days of life.

The last principle is that *overall growth and development occur in spurts, not at a steady rate.* One need only recall the "growing pains" of youth to appreciate the uneven process of physical maturation.

As children develop physically they are also developing mentally. They learn language and social skills largely through social interaction with others in the environment, as they imitate the sounds and gestures of adults and older children. Infants gain information about the world around them by using their senses—hearing, smell, taste, touch, and vision—each of which develops at different periods durng the early months of life. As these senses sharpen and become more sophisticated, so does the infant's ability to extract information from the environment. Eventually, the child begins to integrate his experience and coordinate physical activities accordingly.

I have attempted to summarize a very complex set of events in a few paragraphs. For more detailed information, interested persons can consult the sources listed in the bibliography. Having presented this overview, we will now look at child development for each of the age groups previously examined in terms of child mortality.

PRIOR TO BIRTH: CARE OF THE DEVELOPING FETUS

In order to protect the child effectively, new parents must learn good child care practices. Good infant care begins with the mother taking proper care of herself during pregnancy.

As the fetus (baby in the womb) develops in the uterus, the mother's eating habits, physical activities, and general condition affect its health. While in the womb, the fetus is susceptible to maternal diseases and other conditions that have an impact on the mother's health, as well as a wide array of substances such as alcohol, illegal drugs, and many legal over-the-counter or prescription drugs. Anything the mother consumes can affect her baby's future health. Therefore, it is important that pregnant women talk to their doctors before taking *any* medication. It is equally important that the mother eat proper, balanced meals and take good care of her own health. Cigarette smoking is not only dangerous for the mother, but it can affect her baby's growth and development during pregnancy. It is a practice that should be avoided, at least during the course of the pregnancy. Research has shown that mothers who smoke have a higher incidence of low-birth-weight babies than mothers who do not.

Chapter 2 discussed birth defects and congenital anomalies as persistent causes of death during the first year of life and beyond. The March of Dimes is one of many organizations that support research, health services, and education to prevent birth defects and to help assure a healthy birth for every baby. If parents have questions or need information, these organizations or the family physician can suggest a variety of resources to assist them in their efforts to learn more about and thus avoid birth defects.

We have already talked about how the mother's illnesses can cause birth defects in the child. Therefore, if a woman makes the decision to have a child, she has an obligation to her unborn baby to get good medical care during her pregnancy. She should also be familiar with what will happen to her body during the next nine months so that if something out of the ordinary occurs, she can seek medical attention. When it's time to deliver, proper medical care should be available, and the new infant should be under the care of a physician. New parents need instruction on the many facets of child care. Fortunately, most hospitals and clinics offer child-birth and baby-care classes. Pregnant women, especially first-time mothers, may wish to participate in either or both of these training programs. On the individual level, a woman needs to assume responsibility for her physical well-being during pregnancy, provided she is able. It is the community's moral obligation to see that prenatal care is available to all women whether or not they can afford it.

Since so many mothers of low-birth-weight babies are barely in their teens, we need to make sure this care is where they will use it. Some organizations suggest that prenatal and child-care education be available in high schools, thus allowing teenagers direct access. This makes care more available to the population most in need of it, and not just accessible to those women who can afford it from a private physician. All women must be educated to realize that prenatal care is the first line of defense in the battle to save their developing child. Such available and affordable services are essential if the United States is to make strides in decreasing the number of low-birth-weight babies and, of course, lower its infant mortality rate.

11

Infancy

AN OVERVIEW

In infancy the baby gains about five to seven ounces weekly during the first six months and grows nearly an inch per month during this period. By the time the child has aged six months, its birth weight has roughly doubled. After this first six months, infants gain three to five ounces weekly and grow about one-half inch per month. By the time they have their first birthday, their birth weight has tripled and their body length has increased by 50 percent. At birth, infants breathe through the nose only, but after six months, they are able to breathe through the mouth if the nose is obstructed. During their fourth or fifth month, they begin drooling and teething. At one year of age the chest and head circumferences are about equal.

There is a definite progression of development during the child's first year. In the first month a baby's hands are tightly fisted; objects placed in its hand cannot be held for very long. In these early days of life, the baby's head will fall back if not supported. But by the end of the second month, the infant has attempted to raise its head, can open its hands, and can even move its arms and legs. By four months of age, the child can hold his head erect and can raise his head and chest while lying flat. Before the end of the first three months, the baby has begun to play with his hands; by the sixth month he can grasp objects, and by twelve months he can use a thumb and index finger clumsily to pick up objects. At five months the infant will roll from side to side, and by eight to nine months of age the youngster can sit steady in an upright position.

In just a few more months (at eleven months of age), the child begins to crawl, and at twelve months he can stand alone.

A baby's sensory development follows a pattern also. In the first months the child tolerates minimal frustrations and cries readily to show displeasure. Gazing out at the environment and smiling during the first month are quite common but should not be construed as responses to any specific stimuli. After two months, however, the child will smile in response to a human voice, and the baby's eye will follow objects or a moving person. At two months the cooing begins as the child seems more alert to his surroundings.

By the time infants reach eight months, they cry less, chuckle more, and appear to enjoy making sounds. During this time, babies respond to familiar faces and appear to enjoy being with people. A five-month-old baby can differentiate a parent from a stranger; by six months of age, the youngster will cry in response to a stranger. Between six to eight months of age, babies can make distinct vowel sounds and will imitate others. As infants approach one year, they mimic sounds; respond to their name; show emotions like anger, fear, and love; and will be eager to leave the mother's side and explore the world around them. At twelve months of age babies will experiment with objects and determine their behavior; these infants begin to find alternate ways to achieve tasks.

The parents of an infant must educate themselves regarding the normal growth and development patterns just outlined. They must also make sure that their baby is under the care of a physician and receives regular checkups. Parents need to understand proper nutrition and seek necessary assistance to ensure that their baby eats the proper foods to promote growth and development.

The WIC (Women, Infants, and Children) program is a nutrition and health service that provides mothers with money for purchasing a variety of essential products for themselves and their children. Through its efforts to educate mothers and to supplement the family diet, low-birth-weight problems have been reduced by almost 20 percent. We need more such programs! We also need to ensure through public awareness campaigns that mothers know about the social services available to them and that they are encouraged to participate. Health-care and child-care education programs for our poor children and adults are not adequately funded and are therefore not always nearby or available. If the death toll among the children most at risk is to take a dramatic turn for the better, then every available resource we have must be invested in these young lives. Concerned citizens must vote to protect our infants in their first crucial year of life.

The obvious need for child-care education among new parents is demonstrated by the growing number of accidental drownings in infants less than one month of age, and the increase in accidental deaths for those under one year. We assume common sense will prevail and adults realize that infants should not be left unattended in water—whether it be bath water or the smallest of wading pools—but obviously we have to better educate new parents. Many of these deaths could probably have been prevented if the parents were knowledgeable about safety measures for infants. Also, parents who are familiar with child growth, development, and behavior can be more alert to the signs of illness, disability, or infection in their infants. Good preventive medical care must be available when the child is well, and especially when illness strikes.

WHAT PARENTS CAN DO TO PROTECT INFANTS

Parents need to know the normal range of the growth stages in infants— when a child should begin to roll over, sit up, creep, crawl, and walk— so that proper protective measures can be taken to prevent accidents and injuries that occur most frequently in infants under one year of age. For example, an infant should never be left on any high surface without adult supervision. Though dressing tables and cribs usually have siderails or safety belts, they can only protect a child if they are used. Too many children at this young age die as a result of falls, even from what would appear to be very short heights. Infant seats should not be left on high surfaces if the baby is unattended. Stairways should be blocked with an appropriate safety gate. If an infant is in a high chair, the safety strap should be used. The best rule is never to turn away from an infant on an unprotected surface higher than the floor. It only takes a few seconds for disaster to take its toll.

We also need to ensure that child-care products meet safety standards and have features that adequately protect the infant. It is important to look at packaging and to pay close attention to the age for which the toy or product was designed and developed. Toys should not have small pieces or removable parts. Avoid purchasing stuffed animals with glued-on eyes and noses. Be sure to remove any ribbons around the head or neck of these stuffed toys. To avoid lethal injuries in infants we must make sure they are watched at all times and not placed in jeopardy by leaving them unattended even for short periods without appropriate protection.

When in the bathtub infants should never be left alone. Even an older infant who is capable of sitting unattended can slip and drown in very shallow water.

Infants should sleep in their own bed and not in bed with an adult. If the infant is in a crib, make sure the crib is safe and that the mattress is at least two to three feet below the rail. (Remember my own experience with my nine-month-old daughter.) Make sure older cribs do not have sharp edges and that they are painted with lead-free material. Crib rails should lock securely and the slats should not be more than 2⅜ inches apart so that an infant cannot slide through or stick his head through the slats. Pillows are unnecessary and should never be used; the danger of suffocation is just too great. Do not put infants to bed if they are wearing a bib or any object, such as a pacifier or toy, with a string. Initially the risk of choking is the primary concern, but strings can also catch on crib posts and strangle an infant. I recently read a story about a child who was strangled to death by a crib gym. Inspect these items carefully; perhaps the best practice is to use them only if parents can supervise.

Be on the lookout for small objects on the floor and in other locations. Keep all harmful substances, plants, and electrical objects away from children to avoid accidents, suffocation, and poisonings. Keep the number for the Poison Control Center next to the phone. When in automobiles, infants should always be in an approved safety seat. Allstate Insurance reports that one-third of all infant car seats are not used properly. According to this same source, a safety seat improves a child's chances of surviving an accident by 70 percent. An American Academy of Pediatrics pamphlet outlining proper safety features is available from Allstate Insurance Company (see Appendix A for the address). Allstate recommends that parents (1) fasten the harness snugly over the child's shoulders, (2) select a seat appropriate for the child's weight, (3) face the seat in the proper direction, (4) thread the car's seatbelt through the child's seat properly, and (5) check to see that the seat certifies that it meets federal safety standards. Some police departments have spare safety seats that they will lend to parents for a time, and some states even have a system where the seats can be provided to low-income families who might not otherwise be able to afford them. Parents should consult their local police for information and advice.

Another infant health problem we've discussed is "crib death" or Sudden Infant Death Syndrome (SIDS), a mystifying danger placing many of our youngest citizens in jeopardy. This type of death, because it is so sudden, can be devastating to a family. The National Sudden Infant Death Syndrome Foundation has chapters throughout the country. They have parent support groups, resource materials, and a network of volunteers and professionals ready to help families who have lost a child to SIDS or who want to learn more about this silent killer. The cause of SIDS remains unknown; much research needs to be done to help reduce this unpredictable and as yet unpreventable threat to our infant population. We need to support efforts for research on SIDS because it is the leading cause of death in infants over the age of twenty-eight days.

Infants need adequate nutrition because their growth rate is so rapid. Those who do not receive proper nutrition may fail to thrive (both physically and mentally), or they may develop iron-deficiency anemia. Nutritional needs should be discussed with a physician or nurse and information given to low-income mothers to help them to augment their own diet as well as their child's. This is especially true for expectant mothers as well as those who have delivered and are breast-feeding. An adequate diet, plenty of fluids, and ample rest are essential. If the mother bottle-feeds, she needs to use a formula specifically recommended by a pediatrician. Usually an infant requires supplemental vitamins/nutrients as recommended by the doctor. While feeding the child, mothers should never prop the baby with its bottle because of the potential danger that fluid will enter the lungs. And remember, babies need water in addition to formula for good hydration. Solid foods should not be given to a very small infant without the recommendation of a pediatrician. Each new food should be added separately so any intolerance is easily identified. Babies should never be given homogenized or skim milk because it does not contain all the essential nutrients a young baby needs. Using it instead of breast milk or infant formula can result in nutritional deficiencies.

Parents should be aware of the physical signs of illness. For example, every baby spits ups at times but spitting up large amounts after every feeding may be a reason to consult a physician. Fever, diarrhea, and irritability may also indicate illness. Infants must have their temperature taken rectally rather than orally. Parents should seek advice on how to perform this procedure correctly. Upper respiratory infections are another common source of infant illness. Again, parents should consult their pediatrician for advice when they observe these types of symptoms.

Infants must be kept clean, dry, and warm. Hygiene is important to prevent infection. Safety and hygiene are critical factors for good health during infancy. Close attention just to these fundamental areas can prevent many deaths.

Infants under the age of one year are truly dependent creatures. They rely on adults to meet every physical and emotional need. Unless the adult is prepared to meet these needs the baby will not thrive. Emotionally, the infants feel they are one with the world. As they develop during the first year, they begin to "feel" their difference and then slowly distinguish "self" from those around them. If they are touched with love and affection, this helps them to establish healthy relationships with others in later life. Infants need cuddling and security. If an infant is neglected or touched with anger, the child's development may well be adversely affected. Infants can literally die of neglect—whether it be emotional neglect, physical neglect, or both. Cuddling and touching help all the senses to develop. Parents and adults must remember that human contact and touch are as essential to a baby's growth as are the more basic needs of nourishment and cleanliness.

Certain types of behavior in the infant may indicate a problem and thereby warrant special attention. If the baby seems jittery, irritable, or cries a lot, and this problem persists over a period of time, the child may need medical attention. When the baby doesn't eat, has trouble sleeping, isn't playful, and/or doesn't seem to be gaining weight, a parent should be concerned and seek medical advice. These kinds of behavioral changes may signal physical or emotional problems that should be discussed with and treated by a pediatrician.

Babies are not considerate of their parents' needs. When they cry they are expressing their discomfort. Some parents may not understand this: they become impatient as the crying continues, more distressing and disruptive than ever. Unlike older children who can learn from attempts to correct their behavior, babies can't or shouldn't be punished; they simply lack an adequate level of understanding. If parents find themselves unable to cope, or if they see other adults/parents who cannot handle a baby's normal demands and in desperation resort to physical punishment, everything possible must be done—immediately—to protect that child. If you or someone you know has difficulty coping with an infant and there is suspicion or danger of abuse, don't hesitate—call the child-abuse "hot line" or Parents Anonymous in your community (numbers are listed in Appendix A), an organization that offers confidential help to parents who are at risk of abusing their children. If the child is hurt or in real danger, do not hesitate to contact the local child-protective services or a child-abuse community hot line, as well as the local police. In addition, parents who leave their children in the care of others should always be observant of their child's physical and emotional well-being and question any and all injuries no matter how insignificant.

It is beyond the scope of this book to attempt to teach parents how to differentiate symptoms that are major sources of concern from those that are less potentially lethal. My advice is simple—consult your doctor. Babies ought to be under the care of a physician from birth; and during the child's early life, parents should actively seek the guidance of health-care providers concerning infant care.

WHAT THE COMMUNITY CAN DO

To protect and save those of our children who are not yet born or who are under one year of age, parents and concerned adults should take the following steps:

1. Ensure that mothers receive good medical care during pregnancy to reduce the number of babies who die from low birth weight.

2. Avoid—and teach others to avoid—alcohol, drugs, and cigarette smoking during pregnancy.

3. Use—and encourage every mother to use—all available health-care services for their children. As citizens, we need to ensure that adequate health care and health education are available to all parents.

4. Prepare ourselves and, as much as possible, all mothers—especially teen mothers—for the physical and emotional demands of parenting. If we are to reduce child abuse and neglect, proper health education and parenting classes are needed.

5. Be aware ourselves, and ensure that all mothers are aware, of normal health-care needs, physical growth, and emotional development during early childhood. Infants must be carefully monitored to identify problems before fatal consequences from illness or disease occur.

6. Provide financial and volunteer support to groups and organizations like the March of Dimes and the National Sudden Infant Death Syndrome Foundation so they can continue their vital role in health education and research related to care during pregnancy, infant disability, and reducing the number of infant deaths.

7. Ensure that our infants are protected from accidents that result in fatal injury. These young ones are especially vulnerable to falls and injuries involving automobiles. We need to use proper safety devices to protect them and we must closely supervise their activities at all times. Support is needed for legislation that encourages the

highest standards of safety for products used on or by infants. We must also ensure that current laws passed to safeguard the lives of our children are diligently enforced.

12

Children Aged One to Fourteen

As with infants, parents should be aware of the normal growth and de-velopment patterns of their children at every age. Toddlers are still babies but they are often extremely curious as they walk and climb to explore the unknown. Toddlers imitate their parents, begin to talk, and still put almost everything they can grasp into their mouths. As one mother said of her two-year-old son, "He's into everything." Emotionally, toddlers are willing to explore their environment when mother or a caretaker is close by. They may have objects like a doll, a blanket, or their own thumb to calm them, help them feel secure, or to accompany them while sleeping. Toddlers love to play, and oftentimes they exhibit a wide variety of emo-tions. These youngsters can sometimes run wild, while their parents feel completely incapable of controlling them. Discipline is difficult because reasoning with a child so young often doesn't work. Instead, a parent should give clear instructions and let the child know the immediate consequences of a behavior. Above all, parents need to be consistent in setting forth the rules they impose.

There are certain emotional behaviors for which a parent should consult a pediatrician. All toddlers may exhibit these behaviors but, again, if they persist, attention to the problem is required. For example, children may have difficulty in separating from their parents in secure, nonstressful situ-ations. When a child seems either out of control most of the time or entirely too passive, quiet, and withdrawn—two extremes—a doctor should be consulted. A lack of interest in playing may prove significant, especially since this activity generally consumes the largest part of a small child's day. Parents should also consider talking to their doctor or health professional if the child experiences persistent difficulty in falling asleep. Sometimes when a potty-trained child begins again to soil himself frequently, an emotional or physical disturbance may be the root cause. Spanking and physical punishment do not help in any of these situations, especially if there are underlying physical or emotional problems.

As a preschooler (two to five years) the child's vocabulary increases. He has greater muscle coordination, is much more social in terms of play, and enjoys new-found skills immensely. During the school years before adolescence, he continues to grow, enjoys interaction with peers, and learns the need for rules, but physical changes seem to occur at a slower pace than in the preschool years. It is during this time that many early values begin to form. The period between infancy and adolescence is a time when the child's outside world expands very rapidly. Parents must often try to strike a balance between protecting the child and letting him explore his world.

Preadolescent children feel good about accomplishments. They have wild imaginations and act out very dramatic scenes using toys and other objects. As with infants, parents of younger, preadolescent children can find many resources to help them make decisions about what their children should be allowed to do and how they should be guided. In addition, parents and other interested adults should be concerned if a child consistently exhibits either excessively timid and passive or angry and aggressive behavior. A child with serious physical or emotional problems may have significant difficulties eating and sleeping, in addition to which he might experience bedwetting and have recurring discipline problems in school. Parents should consult their pediatrician or school counselor about these problems and solicit advice on any behaviors about which they have questions. The presence of physical and/or emotional problems may indicate that the child needs professional attention.

Physically, toddlers from infancy to school age change a great deal. They gain bladder and bowel control at about eighteen months. All body systems are well developed with the exception of the reproductive and endocrine (hormone producing) systems. They also have all their temporary teeth. Between the ages of three and five, children experience an annual weight gain of four to six pounds; a two- to two-and-a-half-inch growth rate is not unusual. By four years of age young children walk, squat, run, and learn to jump; they can even ride a tricycle. At the age of three they can usually feed themselves and are speaking in three-to-four-word sentences. Between the ages of two and three, children begin to separate more readily from parents and will engage in play with other youngsters.

By the time a child is five years old, he can usually dress himself, seems to understand the concept of time, and has a larger vocabulary. Children at this age rely on parents for security and reassurance. By the age of seven they have some permanent teeth and weigh close to fifty pounds; they participate in group play and usually begin to tell time.

At age eight or nine a child can bathe without aid and continues to grow approximately two inches each year. He also fully comprehends time and enjoys exploring the neighborhood with friends. He is usually well behaved.

When I look back on all the ages I lived through with my own children, the period between eight and nine is my favorite. My children seemed so willing to please, and were amenable to most things. Personally, I wish I had spent more time teaching and cultivating values during those years. This was the age when they were most receptive, and I probably could have impressed them with specific points more easily than in the teenage years. I could have anticipated some of the problems manifested later by laying the groundwork when it was still possible to tell them something and have them listen.

By twelve years of age, a child's growth in height slows and all remaining permanent teeth emerge. Changes associated with puberty may begin about this time. These kids are capable of abstract thought and—most important for parents—they begin to use the telephone. My advice is to get them their own line! Friends are very important in this age.

Between the ages of thirteen and fifteen, changes resulting from puberty are evident in both sexes. These older children have much more complex reasoning capabilities and seem less involved in family affairs, as they become far more involved in a peer group and with the opposite sex.

WHAT PARENTS CAN DO TO PROTECT THESE CHILDREN

Preventing Accidents

As we discussed earlier, accidental injuries and violence are the primary causes of death among young children. In the 1980s, motor vehicle fatalities and other accidental injuries, including fires and drowning, were the most prevalent external causes of death at ages one to four years and five to nine years. As of 1987, accidents were still the most frequent cause of death in these age groups. The incidence of injuries seems to vary with race and sex. Although no differences associated with these factors were apparent with passenger-related motor vehicle accidents, pedestrian-related accidents and drownings were higher for males. Deaths from fires and homicides were higher for African-Americans than for white children.

The toddler, the preschooler, and the school-age child are very active and prone to accidents and injuries. As parents, the best way to decrease child fatalities from injuries is to make decisions that lessen the likelihood of their occurrence. To safeguard against accidents in which the victim is a young passenger in an automobile, children, like infants in most states, ought to be placed in an approved safety seat. This seat should be used to secure children up to a weight of about forty to fifty pounds. Thereafter, they should use a safety belt and/or other devices with specific accommodations for size. Since safety devices and regulations vary from state to state, parents and concerned adults are advised to consult the local police for information regarding the laws specific to a given area. It is important for parents to realize that children are easily injured or killed in auto accidents; even in minor fender benders, small children unprotected by special seats or lap/shoulder restraints risk becoming projectiles propelled forward in the car or through a window. On impact these youngsters can sustain major physical damage and many die. Some reports indicate that 80 to 90 percent of childhood deaths related to automobile accidents could have been prevented if the youngsters had just been placed in safety devices.

Steps can also be taken to prevent fatal bicycle accidents involving automobiles or those dangerous situations in which a young pedestrian is killed in traffic. As responsible adult drivers, we must realize that children often dart out into the street at any moment at the slightest provocation. Driving cautiously, especially in areas where children are known or suspected to be playing, is a must. As I was working on this chapter, an event occurred that supports the point I have just made.

I was on my way home from the store when a small girl, maybe three or four years of age, caught my eye at the end of my block. She was trotting toward the end of her driveway, as my car approached the front of her house. Her mother was on the front lawn no more than twenty feet from the child, and she yelled for her daughter to stop. I didn't think the little girl would stop, so I brought the car to a complete halt. In fact, the child ran right out into the street in front of my car. If I hadn't anticipated the potential danger of the situation, I might have hit and possibly even killed her. The mother had a lot more confidence in the child's obedience to her commands than I did.

Never overestimate your child's reaction to danger or obedience to your commands. Parents and supervising adults should carefully examine whether or not the children in their care are conscious of potential danger and mature enough to know the hazards of traffic. Can the children cross the street by themselves? Do they understand crossing signals? Are there crossing guards at corners to help them? Do they know they should cross at corners and not cut between parked cars? We often assume that a child has mastered these basic safety rules; but we must constantly reinforce rules about walking and riding bicycles near traffic. We should take the time to really observe that our children have the awareness to cross streets unsupervised and to walk to school or to a friend's house by themselves.

I'll always remember the day my father took time off from work to walk me to school. There was no busing available to my .home, and my parents could not afford a car. My mother had several smaller children and was willing to walk me back and forth, but she was findng it more and more difficult. She had to bundle up all the other smaller kids and make the trip to and from the school twice each day. Naturally, I wanted to walk the distance by myself. The day my father went with me was memorable because he watched me, tested me, and instructed me all at the same time. That simple activity was very effective and I never needed any supervision from that day forward: the lessons and safety rules learned during that walk have remained with me always.

It may take more time these days to teach a child since traffic is heavier, but this effort can save a child's life. Take this time to assess your children's abilities. Teach them and observe that they listen to your instructions. Very small children and toddlers should not be allowed to play near the street and should not be left under the supervision of anyone but an adult if they are playing in an area with easy access to the street, most particularly if it is necessary at any time to cross a street. And if you are watching a group of children, make sure you don't make the mistake of assuming that they will stop running because you yell for them to do so. When you walk with a child make sure you hold his or her hand securely— never allow a small child to cross the street without holding your hand. Discourage older children from "horsing around" while they cross the street. Many of these measures will seem to be just a matter of common sense, but children cannot be relied on to practice common sense.

Youngsters who have bicycles should be familiar with the rules for safe biking. The bike itself should be in good operating condition: proper brakes, a light for night riding, adequate tire pressure, etc. Teach your child the safety rules of bicycle riding and reinforce their importance from time to time. Some police departments hold bike-safety programs at schools or youth organizations. A quick call to your local police station can identify the location nearest you. Adult drivers should exercise caution around young bicyclists: never assume that the child on a bike will react reasonably. *You* must be the one to act prudently.

All-terrain vehicles (ATVs), motorcycles, and other motorized recreational vehicles are potentially very dangerous. My neighbor's child died as a result of an accident involving a mini-bike. When a death from one of these vehicles occurs, it heightens our awareness that these "toys" are extremely dangerous. In my neighborhood, they remain very popular with preadolescents. These kids ride them on large, open flat fields in the summertime. They jump off ramps and speed through wild shrubbery totally unsupervised. Some of these youngsters don't even wear helmets. I'm not attacking the marketing of these toys, but I sometimes wonder if kids have the maturity to "play" with such vehicles in a manner that does not risk fatal injury. Such recreational vehicles do produce their fair share of fatalities.

Skateboarding can be dangerous, too. Many towns and cities are no longer allowing children to play with these toys in the street because of the increase in accidents and injuries when skateboarders mix with automobiles on the road.

Guarding against Poisoning

Poisonings, as we have learned, are a frequent cause of accidental death in young children. Household cleaners and toxic substances should be locked up or placed high enough so that a small child cannot reach them. Medications should never be within easy reach. Most medications now have "childproof" caps, but this is no guarantee that a clever child won't remove the lid from a deadly drug. If a child swallows a dangerous substance, get help immediately. Antidotes for poisons are usually mentioned on the bottle. If you must take the child to an emergency room, or if you call 911 for rescue service, take the suspected container with you and show it to the health-care workers. There are poison-control centers that can be contacted if the antidote is not specified or if it is a medication. Keep the number for the Poison Control Center posted by your phone.

Choking

Foreign objects becoming lodged in the throat is not an uncommon problem confronting the parents of younger children. A toddler finds a penny or a bright bead and instinctively puts it in his mouth. The risk that the child's air passage could become clogged is very real. The American Heart Association and the American Red Cross offer programs that teach interested persons how to save a choking child. The technique used to dislodge the object would depend on the age of the child. However, it is imperative that emergency help be found immediately in case your efforts to dislodge the object, using one or more of the approved methods, fail.

Drowning

Since drownings are also a frequent cause of death in young children, we must make sure that all children learn how to swim and are aware of water safety rules. The Red Cross and YM(W)CA conduct programs to teach swimming, as do some school districts and public pools. No inexperienced child should be allowed to venture near a body of water without at least the benefit of adult supervision and a life preserver.

Backyard pools should be completely fenced in, have self-latching gates, and should not be readily accessible to toddlers and very young children. Even though there are regulations in some areas regarding appropriate pool safeguards, you need to protect your own child. Gates and doors can be left open; a young child could wander into the pool area, fall into the water unnoticed, and drown. Public pools should always have trained lifeguards, and older children should never swim alone. They should always swim in a supervised area.

In addition, the danger of drowning can be equally real in nonswimming situations. Very young children are at risk of drowning in bath water or any large container where water might collect (e.g., water barrels, small fountains, ponds in the yard, etc.) or be used for household chores. Just recently, there have been news stories about the number of small children who play around large buckets of water used for cleaning. A child leans over into the bucket to play with the water or to retrieve a toy and topples over headfirst into the container. Once inside, the child cannot get out and ultimately drowns.

Fire Safety

Fires also claim many young lives. Children must learn at an early age that matches and lighters are not toys and should not be touched. If parents find their child's infatuation with matches to be a persistent problem, they should seek the help of a counselor. Typically, the young persistent firesetter is male. Some theories suggest that this signifies the presence of an unsatisfied need for companionship or the desire to seek revenge against some significant person. Counseling is the first line of defense. Parents should make sure that matches and lighters are not within easy reach. Fire-related deaths in children are relatively high in the one-to-four age group. To these children, a cigarette lighter seems an ideal toy: it's colorful, small enough to handle, and it makes "pretty sparks." But it's a dangerous toy: almost eight thousand fires are started each year by small children.

Parents should also make sure that they review with their children what to do in the event of a fire. Fire drills at home are excellent preparation. All homes and apartments should have a functioning smoke detector. These devices are not only inexpensive but they can save precious lives. In some cities, the generous donations of caring people have made it possible for city fire departments to provide poor families with smoke detectors free of charge.

Make sure your home does not have obvious fire hazards, such as overloaded electrical plugs or collections of flammable substances or rags. Ensure that small children have flame-retardant clothing and pajamas. Parents should have a fire extinguisher in the home if possible and should be familiar with how to put out small fires. Parents and adults should be aware that many children lose their lives each year because an adult fell asleep while smoking.

All adults should know basic principles of fire safety and should make sure their children learn them. Many local fire departments offer adult programs and sponsor fire-safety exhibits for school children. However, the important responsibility for fire prevention lies with parents and other adults. Our school buildings and our homes must be fire safe and properly equipped with smoke detectors. Parents should know how to respond quickly if a fire starts, and of course parents should not invite disaster by leaving small children unattended at home. All too often we hear news reports about children who have died during a tragic blaze in a house with no adult or parent present.

Firearms Safety

Accidental shootings are becoming a more prevalent problem in youngsters aged one to fourteen. Young children, who are inexperienced with the handling of firearms, should never have access to them: to maintain safety, these weapons should always be kept in a locked cabinet. It's hard to believe that people would leave a loaded pistol or gun where a child could reach it, let alone play with it like a toy. Regrettably, the negligence of parents and other adults provides far too many opportunities for fatal injuries. Additionally, parents who have guns in the house should ensure that their children are well aware of the dangers of firearms.

My father was an avid hunter. There were handguns and rifles in a cabinet at home but it was always locked and the ammunition was never in close proximity to his children. When we were older and more mature, my brothers and I were enrolled in National Rifle Association programs before we were ever permitted to handle a gun or to accompany my father hunting. In our house, we were never allowed to aim a gun—not even a toy replica—directly at ourselves or another person without inviting reprisal. I've long since lost any desire to hunt or to handle guns, but I still know how to handle one safely. Again, take the time to teach your child about the dangers of guns.

Confronting Child Abuse and Neglect

Another major threat to our toddlers and school-age children is that posed by the many forms of violent death. Of all the violence perpetrated on children, the most offensive is parental abuse and/or neglect. Some reports indicate that almost one million children are abused annually. According to Senator Paula Hawkins's book, *Children at Risk,* men, especially live-in boyfriends, are the major in-home abusers. Other information indicates that mothers abuse children most often. However, when abuse becomes fatal, there is usually a man responsible (Hawkins, 1986). These live-in boyfriends are often not accustomed to dealing with young children, but they serve as an inexpensive alternative to safe day care or babysitters in situations where mothers cannot watch their own children. Irritation and frustration resulting from the child's behavior many times results in child abuse and/or severe injuries. Therefore, young mothers should be wary of leaving a small child with someone who may be inexperienced at coping with that child's behavior. Certainly, this abuse is not just delivered by men or live-in boyfriends. Mothers, babysitters—anyone—can be a child abuser.

Parental abuse is caused by a variety of factors, one of the most significant is that abusive parents have often been abused children themselves. Parents who feel they cannot cope with the demands of being a parent should call a community assistance hotline or talk with their doctor, a social worker, or an agency representative committed to helping with this problem. Parents Anonymous, an organization committed to reducing child abuse, will provide parents with confidential help if they call the group's hotline. They also have parent support groups that can be most helpful in treating the abuser. For a parent or other adult to admit that a problem exists is difficult to be sure, but it's far better than fatally injuring or killing your own or someone else's child in a fit of rage. Other factors contributing to child abuse are poverty, divorce, fighting between parents, and drug or alcohol dependency on the part of a parent, to name just a few. The most an adult can do to prevent death related to child abuse is to seek help for personal abusive tendencies, and to report suspected abuse to the proper authorities. Don't mind your own business if you witness child abuse! *Report it!* If you have contact with children who are afraid of parents at home, show evidence of repeated injuries, or exhibit some of the abnormal behaviors for their age group (as we discussed earlier), perhaps there is abuse.

Society must work together to find solutions to the problems that breed child abuse. All concerned citizens must help change laws that protect abusers and make sure that the penalties for abuse and murder are more harsh. Government and law enforcement at all levels should keep better, more centralized records of abuse, all of which are confidential but are not destroyed when charges are dropped. One social worker told me that she had investigated a report of child abuse, but normal investigation procedures failed to demonstrate any evidence of abuse. The charges of abuse were subsequently dropped and all records were expunged. A year later the child was found dead. The murder has been attributed to the live-in boyfriend. He was present during the initial investigation as well.

We also need to consider abused child assistance programs such as the one at the New York Foundling House. This program, developed by Dr. Victor Fontana, has been successful in providing services to abused children and their parents. Another such program, Child-Haven in Washington State, offers comprehensive treatment and enrichment for abused children and their parents. These facilities may serve as a model for programs in your own community. To locate educational programs on effective parenting that can help adults deal with children and their behavior, and for appropriate counseling resources, contact your church, synagogue, local school, or the child protective services agency in your community. In addition to making sure that community help is readily available, we must work with local authorities to assure that the services offered to prevent child abuse are effective.

Violence against young children, as we all know, can also come from strangers. There is an increasing number of missing children in this country.

Many times noncustodial parents abduct their own children. Additionally, some children come to great harm at the hands of unknown, violent adults. Grace Hechinger in her book *How to Raise a Street Smart Kid* suggests that parents can initiate practical steps to reduce the chances that their children will be abducted and/or physically harmed. One such method is for the parents to make sure that they know where their child is at all times and that they do not leave their child alone in the car, the yard, a store, or any other place. She suggests that parents avoid putting nametags on their child's books and clothing; this prevents would-be abductors from being on a first-name basis with a child. Parents and concerned adults should make sure that children know their own home phone number and are familiar with their neighborhoods, especially what to do if they happen to get lost. Parents must always be familiar with their child's habits, friends, special places, etc. Be sure to have recent photos (taken every six months), and know where the child's dental and medical records are in case they are needed. Some communities have suggested that children be fingerprinted. Apparently this is a source of much debate; however, a call to the local police station should provide information about this alternative and how to start such a program in your community. For older children, a good alternative talked about in the literature is the neighborhood "safe" house. Children can go to these houses when they need help or when they are bothered by strangers. Some communities have such programs and they do provide a protective mechanism for older children who do not play in the immediate vicinity of their homes. Other precautions that prove helpful include making a videotape of your child; this can be useful in the event that your son or daugher is missing, runs away, or is lost. If your child is missing or lost, call the police and be aware of organizations that can help. If your child is a runaway, there are agencies that can provide support and counseling. In recent years, a national computer network linking law enforcement agencies has been developed. This allows much more effective communication of local police departments with the FBI. (A number of the private and public organizations that can be called in connection with missing or runaway children are listed in Appendix A.)

As with parental abuse, if you suspect that your child has been abused by a friend, neighbor, family member, or stranger, do not ignore the problem. Get immediate help from local child protection agencies, the social services department, or the police or sheriff's department.

Providing Good Child Care

As adults, we should make every effort to see that there are adequate resources for child care. If good, affordable day care or babysitting were available, children would not be left with people who are unprepared to look after them properly. Young mothers must be taught to be wary of leaving their child in the hands of inexperienced caretakers or those who are not emotionally capable of dealing with the child's behavior.

There are various options for child care and parents should consider them fully before choosing the one that best suits their needs. It must be acknowledged, however, that these choices are *not* available to all parents. Therefore, we must, in addition to taking good care of our own children, ensure that care alternatives for children are available to all mothers and that they are of the highest quality and reasonably priced. For those mothers who cannot afford child care, either publicly provided or funded care must be made available.

Child care in the home is a good alternative especially if the child is an infant or toddler; in these early years they have less need for social play and they do receive more direct attention to their needs with a babysitter in familiar surroundings. Toddlers desire more individual contact with a loving adult than do older children, who like playing with kids their own age. A parent may just need someone for a child who requires supervision before and after school. Having someone in the home may work especially well when both parents have jobs and are not always able to get home on time. Some possible alternatives to a sitter might be relatives or a neighborhood teenager. However, the neighbor or teenager must be someone who is known and has demonstrated competence in caring for children. To determine this ask for references from other parents or neighbors for whom the person has worked. It is also a good idea to have the sitter visit while your child is present so that you can observe how the person deals with your youngster. In addition, make sure that you are very clear about the sitter's responsibilities with regard to the child: those who care for your child should become very familiar with the infant or toddler as well as his care and safety.

There are even reputable firms that provide "live-in nannies." If you can afford these services, they may be an alternative. For most parents, it's far more practical and sensible to find someone who will look after their child while they are away. Sometimes there may be a mother in the neighborhood who takes care of several children during the day. A group of mothers can form a co-op and help one another with child-care needs. The advantage to these alternatives might be that the mother who provides these services has children of her own who can play with the child being looked after. Preschoolers and school-age kids really enjoy these opportunities to play with other children. Another attractive feature of in-house or co-op day-care centers is that they are often closer to home. Of course, there are day-care centers that operate for profit (some of which are affiliated with large franchises or private organizations), nonprofit community or church-funded day-care centers, or services provided by an employer (least often)—many of which provide services for even very young infants. Some schools and organizations provide after-school programs for children who need supervision until the parent returns from work. Other children may spend their after-school hours at home alone or with older brothers and sisters. However, most experts believe that a child under ten years of age should not be left alone after school.

With these choices, the safety and welfare of our children must come first. No matter where the child care is provided—at home, at a neighbor's home, or in a day-care facility—it is important to know that the structure is childproof. Are there electrical outlet protectors? Are the cabinets that store dangerous objects or substances securely locked? If the child will be cared for at a neighbor's home, is *that* home clean and safe? Does it appear to be a place where your child will be stimulated and happy?

These criteria hold true for selecting any day-care provider. A safe, clean environment should be sought where the child will be happy. Parents should be familiar with the fees charged for services rendered, whether the care provider can properly look after children when they are ill, the hours that services are available, and what procedures are in place in the event that emergencies arise. Do take the time to observe the activities in a day-care center. Stay involved and interested in your child's program and be alert for signs of any abnormal distress. If your child is in day care, the facility should be licensed or registered according to all local and state regulations and the director should have a solid background in early childhood education. You should be able to visit and observe your youngster at any time. The people who are employed at the facility should be warm and caring and there should be enough help to ensure that your child gets the kind of attention a developing young mind and body needs. The facility should have access to medical help for an emergency. All child-care providers should be trained in how to provide emergency care to a choking child or to a child who is not breathing. Above all, observe and listen to your child; you can pick up on problems that become apparent no matter which alternative is chosen.

If your children must care for themselves at home (if they are what has come to be called latchkey children), show them what to do in the event of a fire; review fire safety rules and have regular fire drills. Instruct children in what to do if they return home and suspect that a burglary has taken place. They should not enter the house but go to a neighbor, to the police, or even back to school and get help. Make sure your children know how to handle phone calls in your absence (so they don't alert callers to the fact that they are alone), and that they never permit anyone to enter the house while they are alone. Make sure that any other safety procedures you have put in place are reviewed and that the children call you to check in when they arrive home from school. You should also have a number that they can call in the event that help is needed, and of course the children should know how to use or have access to all emergency numbers (police, fire, poison center, doctor, etc.). Many communities have programs for latchkey kids: some organizations have volunteers who call to make sure that the children are all right in the home. Many cities throughout the United States have educational programs specifically geared to latchkey kids. Parents and the children receive instruction on how best to cope with their situation. In the meantime, reinforcing safety and emergency procedures in children who must care for themselves is essential if we are to prevent fatal accidents. Investigate the latchkey programs in your area. (There is a number in Appendix A that you can call to obtain more information.)

Recently, my sister Kate secured a full-time job and my ten-year-old niece, Ellen, had to look after herself for about thirty minutes between leaving school and her mother's arrival home from work. My twenty-two-year-old daughter, Amanda, is very close to her cousin, and one afternoon I heard the two of them talking on the phone. Amanda was telling Ellen that she shouldn't mention anything to people about her mother not being home; Amanda carefully instructed Ellen on how to handle the phone while her mother was in transit. It had been almost twelve years since I gave that speech to Amanda. It really made an impression.

Knowing the Warning Signs of Potential Suicide

Self-inflicted violence or suicide is a growing problem among teenagers but is also in evidence with children in the younger age groups we have been discussing. Children particularly at risk are those who suffer from low self-esteem. We must face the facts about childhood stress. The world is a very hard place for children. It can make them feel very insecure about themselves. One of the reasons kids are under more stress is that in many homes both parents work, which leaves a lot less time for family sharing and guidance. Divorce and the fact that many children are in single-parent homes put added pressure on the usual stress of growing up. Some parents may be superachievers who push hard for their children to excel academically or in other activities. Our culture has become intensely sexualized and drug-oriented, forcing kids to face these issues and make decisions at an early age. When a child feels bad for a long period of time, his self-esteem suffers, and when this happens he could be in danger. Parents need to consider and actively combat these stresses. We must do everything we can to encourage, reinforce the positive aspects of childhood, and make kids feel good about themselves.

Drug and alcohol abuse are more prevalent in teenagers, but involvement in the drug culture poses a significant danger to pre-adolescent children and is becoming more obvious every day. Other precautions parents can take with regard to drugs and alcohol will be discussed when we focus on teenagers, but it is important to mention here that the potential fatalities these drugs can cause shouldn't be ignored in younger children.

Practicing Good Health and Knowing the Danger Signs of Illness

To maximize physical health, parents should instill in their children good values early in life regarding health practices. When children learn at an early age the principles of health promotion and disease prevention, they carry these values with them throughout their lives.

We know that congenital anomalies and neoplasms are responsible for the deaths of many children between the ages of one and fourteen. Good, regular medical checkups are critical to the early detection of health problems. Some congenital anomalies can be readily recognizable at birth, or they might go undetected until much later in life. If parents are alert to physical and mental changes or abnormalities, they are better prepared to get the necessary help for their child and perhaps save the child's life.

I remember driving my son home from the park one day when he was two and a half. When I had dropped him off several hours before, he was all smiles and energy. Now he just sat quietly in his car seat and appeared to be tired. At first this seemed natural after an afternoon of running around in the park. But then I noticed that he looked too pale, too listless. I reached over and put my hand on his head; he felt very warm. I got an uneasy feeling, so instead of going straight home, I decided to drive by the doctor's office. It's a good thing I did. By the time I got half-way there, my son had had a convulsion. When I arrived at the doctor's office, his temperature had soared to 105°. The convulsion was related to this high temperature. A child can get severely ill very quickly. I knew my son's behavior was not normal for him and in this instance I made a correct decision. He had an ear and throat infection and needed antibiotics immediately. This demonstrates how parents should respond to changes in their child's emotional and/or physical behavior. Had I not observed this change or the seizure, my son might have died from that infection.

Besides being attentive to changes in our children's physical behavior and ensuring that they have regular medical care and dental checkups, we should teach them good health practices. Basic hygiene and good nutrition practices not only prevent illness but render children less vulnerable to accidents and problems later on in their teenage years.

I recently had quite an enlightening conversation with a fellow faculty member's four-year-old girl. This child, who is a joy to talk to, told me in her typical animated style that she didn't like a particular type of "fast food" because it was high in "nodium" (sodium) and fat. I realized how aware she was of what she ate. We must create this awareness in all our children.

Physical fitness is also important. Children need exercise appropriate to their age. We know exercise helps develop muscles and bones, and improves attention span and self-reliance, and tends to reduce anxiety. Children can benefit greatly from eating well and vigorous physical exercise.

We discussed briefly how stress can cause behavioral problems in children. Parents can help preschoolers deal with stress by reading to them and through puppet play. For toddlers, consistent, predictable parental behavior and a secure home environment are two of the best ways to reduce anxiety. Stress reduction in older children can be accomplished to a great extent if parents are able to bolster the child's self-esteem. This can be done through projects, games, and discussions that make children feel better about themselves.

A counselor friend of mine, who specializes in pre-adolescents, volunteered that the major problem he encounters in children is this pervasive lack of self-esteeem, which he believes makes them more prone to accidents, suicide, and some physical illnesses. Children who are confident and self-assured can often avoid such behavioral traps as smoking, alcohol, and drugs if they trust themselves and their choices. For our children's health and well-being, we parents should be role models. We must practice what we preach.

Teaching Your Children How to Respond to Emergencies

Parents and concerned adults should cultivate in young people a healthy respect for avoiding environmental hazards. Children should know how to respond to hazardous conditions in the event that they inadvertently are confronted with them. Children should be involved in projects that are health-oriented or that raise their awareness of health issues. This makes them conscious of important health-related issues.

I remember when my son, Henry, was two and my daughter, Amanda, was four; we were watching television one rainy day in my room. I inadvertently had left a book of matches on the night stand. The gate was across the door and they were safe and secure in the room with me—or so I thought. After a time, I dozed off. I awoke to Amanda pounding me about the face and chest to arouse me. Henry had lit the bedclothes. Amanda, alert to the danger of fire even at four, took him across the room and told him to stay there. She then came back to wake me up and got me out of bed. She saved my life and hers, as well as her brother's. She knew fire was *bad*. She didn't hide, but was aware of the danger and acted aggressively in response. I should have known better than to leave matches where they could find them.

On another occasion, when Henry was nine or ten years old, he and his friends were playing in a large wooded area beyond our backyard, where there is a shallow stream. That year, due to a great deal of rainfall, the stream was almost four feet wide and waist-high on my son; the stream-bed was quite muddy and boggy. Even though the water wasn't particularly deep, the streambed was too muddy to support a person's weight.

The boys decided to explore the shore along the water. Henry inadvertently slipped in and, with the softness of the bottom, was quickly immersed almost to his chin. One of his friends panicked and ran off in the direction of home, but the other boy threw a large branch over the width of the stream and told my son to hang on. He came quickly to the house to get me, and I pulled Henry out. I am grateful that one of them kept a cool head. The youngster knew some basic principles, applied them, and immediately got help. Henry remained calm and didn't panic. If he had thrashed about, he might have become more immersed in the water and mud.

On one other occasion, when Henry was three (he was a pip!), he opened the back door and went outside while I was cooking. I quickly noticed that he was gone and went outside in the backyard to search for him. In just that short time, Henry had opened the gate between my yard and my neighbor's. My neighbor, George, was fixing his garage roof and had left a ladder propped up on the side of the building. His ten-year-old son, Phil, noticed Henry climbing the ladder and ran outside just as my boy reached the roof. Phil called his mother, who quickly came out as Phil ran to the ladder. He didn't grab Henry but talked to him while his mother ran next door to get me. As I was coming out of my house, my neighbor stopped me and told me what had happened. Henry was so delighted by this big boy talking so nicely to him that he remained seated. Meanwhile, with Phil's help, I got my son off the roof. I was very impressed with Phil's calm and mature behavior. Not much can compare with seeing your two-year-old on a roof. I never again left the back door unlocked, even if I was in the room. I also applaud my neighbors and their son for the calm, efficient manner with which they handled the emergency.

Children can learn how to protect themselves and assist others who are in danger without putting themselves in jeopardy. I think these experiences illustrate how resourceful children can be if parents are willing to make a major effort to educate young people about safety and proper procedures in emergency situations.

WHAT THE COMMUNITY CAN DO

There are various methods that parents, adults collectively, and communities as a whole can use to decrease childhood fatalities in toddler, preschool, school-age, and pre-adolescent groups. Parents need to explore these methods for their own children and to support efforts to help protect the general welfare of all children:

1. We need good available child care to safeguard our children's health and to detect illness before it proves fatal. Children, when ill, need care before an infection or condition rages out of control.

2. We need to wear safety belts and to ensure that our children do as well. We should also be sure that young children up to a certain size are restrained in an approved car safety seat when they are passengers in any automobile. Parents should never hold, or allow anyone else to hold, a small child or infant while they are passengers in a car. We must ensure that laws protecting child passengers are in place in our community and that they are enforced.

3. When driving we need to be alert to young pedestrians. We should not assume that these children will behave reasonably or prudently to protect their own safety. They are dependent on the adult driver to react and to prevent accidental death.

4. We should not allow children to play unsupervised near traffic, and we should ensure that children know how to cross streets safely before they are allowed to do so on their own. Small children must always cross hand in hand with an adult. We need to make sure that school crossings are always attended.

5. Swimming pools and other bodies of water should not be readily accessible to an unsupervised child. Principles of water safety and swimming instruction should be provided to children as soon as they are capable.

6. Fire prevention and safety measures should be enforced and taught to the community as well as to children, who should be supervised as much as possible. Latchkey kids should be carefully trained to protect themselves when they are alone at home. Parents should have methods in place for children who must be home on their own. Matches and other flammable materials should never be left in easy reach of children. Parents should make sure that their homes are fire safe; that smoke detectors are installed, and that they work. Children should be trained to respond to a house fire with practice fire drills, especially if they are older and spend time alone at home without adult supervision.

7. Child-safety programs on safe bicycling should be a priority both at home and in the community.

8. Child abuse must be monitored and treated before it proves lethal. There must be ready access to counseling for abusers, and adequate foster care available when children have to be removed from their home environment. Parents need to address the problems in their own families, but they must also make sure that programs are in place to help less fortunate children. Concerned adults must ensure that the community organizations and agencies have systems in place to deal with child abuse. Our law-enforcement agencies must have systems in place to deal with missing children, while all of us do what we can for our own children to prevent kidnapping by strangers.

9. Adequate child care must be available when parents are not able to provide direct care themselves. Child care facilities should be safe and comfortable; parents should never have to settle for a particular day-care or child-care alternative. We must strive to make adequate day care a viable, affordable alternative for all parents in this country.

10. The problems that produce childhood injury and death must be attacked from a wide variety of perspectives. We must work to find ways to improve child welfare for the poor and to increase their access to the services that help safeguard the health and well-being of all children.

11. We need education programs that teach parents how to deal effectively with discipline and to care for their children at all ages.

12. Our children must be educated at an early age about drugs and alcohol.

13. We have to provide more organized, comprehensive services to young children who are at high risk for childhood death.

14. We must teach children how to handle emergencies, by showing them how to behave in specific situations without needlessly endangering their own lives.

15. We can help our children by organizing clubs, youth groups, etc. that cultivate self-sufficiency.

13

Teenagers

AN OVERVIEW

Anyone who has raised a teenager will attest that they are a different breed. Their bodies are developed but their minds have not matured to the point where they can completely take charge of their own lives. They resist authority and often have difficulty adjusting to the oncoming demands of adulthood. Teens tend to be very interested in pleasing themselves and often are not aware of the consequences of their actions, either to themselves or to others. They are generally very energetic, enthusiastic, idealistic, and spend a lot of time in activities outside of school. Parents and other adults may experience great difficulty understanding their behavior. The teen years are often turbulent and unpredictable, and many parents suddenly realize they are on one side of the generation gap and their child is on the other. Teenage dress codes, music, recreational activities, entertainment, and values may seem alien to adults. The child's desire to please peers and to gain their acceptance becomes a more pressing issue than pleasing parents. Teenagers take more risks and at times seem to lack any fear of injury or death. They feel invincible. Their adult bodies give them sexual drives, which, when coupled with their lack of perception about the consequences of their actions, can make them vulnerable to pregnancy as well as sexually transmitted diseases. Experimentation with sex can have a lasting impact on their lives if it results in pregnancy and ultimately the birth of a child. Then we have immature adults who haven't completed their own growth and development finding themselves responsible for another tiny, dependent child.

In regard to their growth and development, by the age of fifteen, most boys and girls have grown to their adult height, have become sexually mature, and physically resemble adults. At this point, they have consolidated a sexual identity and may be sexually active. They also attain emotional independence.

In essence, of all the childhood growth and development periods the teen years may be the most difficult. As a parent, the most problematic aspect for me was my utter loss of control. I remember believing that my son and daughter had never been more difficult. At times, they seemed angry and distant. I compensated by trying to hold on to them more tightly because what they said and did sometimes frightened me. I realized they were at risk for many problems even though I cared and was trying as hard as I could to protect them. There were very difficult situations that shook me to the core of my being, and there were times when I thought I would burst with pride because they did something so wonderful.

WHAT PARENTS CAN DO TO PROTECT TEENAGERS

The Importance of a Good Parent-Teen Relationship

Dr. Lee Salk has suggested some strategies to help with the teen-parent relationship. A good relationship with your teenage children can help them make thoughtful decisions about their activities when they are away from your watchful eye and guidance. Developing a good relationship with your teen is easier if you have already established a strong, binding relationship with them at an earlier age. Then you have a foundation on which to build during the rocky times. Dr. Salk suggests listening to them, as well as teaching teens how to weigh the pros and cons of a situation and to make decisions. Parents also need to be tolerant of some "crazy" behaviors—like purple spiked hair, strange clothing trends, unusual uses of language—and not nag and make an issue of them. Spend time with your child; talk about and develop mutual interests. It's important that parents know their children's friends, get to know the parents of those friends, and develop a rapport with teachers and counselors. Within such a network, information can be shared without "prying." It's important to set reasonable limits. Make sure children receive and understand accurate information on sex, alcohol, and drugs. (Some literature that may help parents deal with teen behavior appears in Appendix B.)

For families who have serious problems with teen behavior, there is a nationwide movement called TOUGHLOVE (see Appendix A), which is a community-based method for parents to form their own support group and learn strategies that help themselves and their teens make positive changes.

Based on personal experience with my teenage children, I would urge parents to listen to their kids and try to be attuned to their behavior. I learned to listen when certain things happened to my kids because I ignored or wasn't paying attention to what they said. Consequently, when something negative happened, I knew in my heart there were previous verbal and behavioral cues that I should have heeded. I learned fast that those cues, if ignored, might produce situations that could really harm my children.

I thought of myself as a concerned, caring parent, but I had to develop my observational and listening abilities. I had to "tune in" and keep an open mind. I suddenly found out that there were many things my children and I didn't agree on, but I searched for those things on which we did agree and reestablished our relationship on that foundation.

It also became obvious that I had to be much more flexible. When our values are questioned, we sometimes become more rigid about them. I had to learn to see my values as my children did and at least be willing to look at my beliefs through their eyes. This is very difficult: Some values, thoughts, and attitudes I did not believe I should change, but the fact that I was willing to discuss them openly helped to establish greater mutual trust and rapport. That kind of give and take in the parent-child relationship is very much a part of the teenage years. I do think that a good home life is important, but the environment outside the home can be more problematic especially in the teen years.

The rebellious spirit of youth is normal and often expected for this age group. However, when a child becomes progressively more difficult and uncontrollable, experiences difficulty with friends or trouble in school, and is generally very angry and aggressive over an extended period of time, counseling may be in order. On the other hand, a child may be very withdrawn, depressed, and anxious. This signals distress, too. Either one of these extremes can alert parents to the presence of serious problems with self-esteem. If your teen feels bad about himself/herself, you need to find a way to help. Herbert Wagemaker, in his work *Why Can't I Understand My Kids,* stresses the importance of making children believe that they are okay and that they are worth something. This is especially important during the stress-laden teenage years.

Self-Esteem: The Key to Psychological Well-Being

Teenagers are caught between wanting security and wanting to be independent. This often gives rise to much anger and resentment. Therefore, although they may resent restrictions imposed by parents, they do interpret these simultaneously as an expression of their parents' love and concern. Behavioral limits that are fair, reasonable, and consistent will provide teens with the structure they need to resist peer pressure. The most effective disciplinary strategy is mutual problem solving: areas of concern are discussed and mutually acceptable solutions are developed that maximize the child's independence while easing the parent's concerns. This is a strategy on which both parent and child can agree. Such an approach also demonstrates that the parent trusts the teen, an issue about which teenagers of all age groups are sensitive.

I interviewed a teen counselor, whom I'll call Jack. He emphasized that problems with self-esteem set the stage for many difficulties experienced in the teen years. When a child experiences a severe loss of self-esteem, extremes in behavior are not uncommon. At one end of the spectrum is the child who becomes so totally immersed in the values and actions of the peer group that he or she seems never to be capable of an independent thought or action. At the other end is the kid who drops out and doesn't involve himself with any friends or activities. These teens appear isolated and withdrawn. Jack has noticed that those who immerse themselves in the peer group are more likely to participate in gang or cult-type activity. They also seem more likely to become involved with addictive substances or unlawful activity, especially if these are activities supported and promoted by the peer group. The members lose their identities in such a group.

On the other hand, the isolationist often will have greater suicidal tendencies. Jack also believes that the kids with low self-esteem frequently suffer from a very negative self-image. Females who suffer from negative self-image tend to have a very distorted view of their body. As a result, Jack has seen an increased incidence of the eating disorder known as anorexia nervosa, especially in adolescent females. I asked him to discuss this further; even though this is not a leading cause of death in teens, it may lead to death in the adult years. There is such an emphasis in the media on thin, attractive females that teenage girls dread being fat or being perceived as fat. These females do have a distorted image of their body size and overestimate their dimensions. They go on starvation diets: Some will eat and then induce vomiting (bullimorexia). They may also take laxatives, diuretics, or enemas to eliminate food. These anorexics do not lack appetite; they simply refuse to eat. Jack says the cause for this is unknown but that it usually follows an adolescent crisis, a change due to puberty, or a trauma (like parental divorce).

A close friend of mine who has been in therapy for years for this problem began vomiting after meals at thirteen years of age as a method of weight reduction. This continued until age twenty-four when she finally received therapy. The beginning of her vomiting followed a bitter parental separation. Apparently, her mother and father fought about everything two people could ever fight about after they separated. My friend became a pawn in their pitched battle. She began to feel very bad about herself, and after a time became a full-blown anorexic. If a teen exhibits dramatic weight loss after such a traumatic event, parents should seek counseling for the child immediately.

Jack also says that a lack of parental guidance and love often reduces self-esteem. This reduced self-esteem can set the stage for suicide.

Jack sees self-esteem as the crucial element in all teenage behavioral problems. Runaways often experience this lack of self-esteem as parents fail to give the love and support the child believes is needed. Jack interprets membership in communal-type groups as a method of dealing with real or perceived parental rejection.

To bolster self-esteem this counselor suggests that parents listen to their teenagers; make them aware that parents do care about their feelings, thoughts, and attitudes; reinforce their sense of worthiness; teach them to see their positive qualities; engage in mutual problem solving; convey trust and respect for them as individuals; set reasonable limits and abide by them; and be consistent. Jack thinks that when the child deviates from these mutually agreed-upon norms, parents should allow teens to face the consequences of their actions, not move in to cover for or protect them so they do not have to be accountable.

Parental Attitudes and the Dangers of Alcohol and Substance Abuse

As we noted previously, the number one killer of fifteen to twenty-year-olds is auto accidents involving alcohol. The statistics have shown that this is a major threat to our teenage population. Over four and a half million teenagers between the ages of fourteen and seventeen are problem drinkers. One out of three high-school seniors will get drunk on a weekend. Scary, isn't it? What can parents do to reduce or eliminate this problem?

We have to examine our own attitudes about alcohol. Alcohol is a drug and it is addictive. In a recent article in *Parents* magazine, Mary

Ellen Donovan discusses what a child should know about alcohol abuse. For one thing, according to Ms. Donovon, kids make decisions about alcohol as early as the fifth grade. Parents should discuss with their kids how liquor, wine, and beer advertisements appeal to a person's desire to be attractive and popular.

Our goal as parents should be to prevent problems, not to wait until we know a problem exists and then react to it. We need to make rules about drinking and drug use in the family and spell out the consequences of breaking those rules. Do not assume your male child is more likely to have problems than your female child. New reports indicate that female children are using alcohol almost as much as their male peers.

Above all, listen to your child. Don't give mixed messages. Don't say one thing and do another with respect to alcohol and drugs. It confuses your children and makes them less willing to abide by the rules parents establish. Build your child's self-esteem: Remember, when you're not around, children have to deal with the pressure of friends to "join in." Just saying no is not an option to teenagers who don't feel comfortable with themselves.

Kids from dysfunctional or poor families often are most vulnerable. Their home cannot provide the kind of love and support they need, so being excluded by friends becomes a major concern in their teenage lives.

Education at the school and/or community level is a must to avoid substance-abuse problems. Parents and adults should get involved in making sure that such programs are available to students. They may have to do this through the school board or through the Parent Teachers Association (PTA). The program that is developed should be comprehensive and continuous. It is also suggested that the program involve all school personnel, including nonteaching staff, such as bus drivers and janitors, because many times these individuals develop trusting relationships with students. Such relationships can be vital when a student is in trouble. If these employees know how to handle a problem, they, too, can help find a solution. Whatever the program is, it should rely heavily on parental support and involvement.

Many school districts have such programs in place already. There are communities that offer counseling and support through youth organizations, which perform the same functions as the in-school programs. They can be of great help to parents and students alike. Organizations like Mothers Against Drunk Driving (MADD) and Students Against Drunk Driving (SADD) provide information and/or have local programs based in schools or other locations where there are organized activities related to raising awareness about alcohol abuse, as well as the dangers of driving while intoxicated. The problem of teenage drinking and driving and the resulting deaths is serious enough in any community that adults should organize efforts to educate and provide ways to modify this behavior.

In my community, many types of activities are available during prom nights and other major teen occasions so that kids are given the choice not to get involved with alcohol or drugs. In one suburb, a youth court is in place with a professionally trained counselor to deal with teen alcohol-related driving violations. Still other communities have programs whereby families sign an agreement to restrict the use of alcohol and drugs at social gatherings in their homes. These are called "safe homes" and they provide reasonable nonalcohol and drug-free alternatives for social activities involving teenagers.

Parents should restrict the use of alcohol in their homes. Store owners who sell alcohol to minors should face stiff penalties and imprisonment if there are ongoing violations. Adults of legal age should face penalties and/or fines for buying alcohol for minors. It is important to note that, according to some reports, a very high percentage of our high-school seniors consume alcohol regularly even though it is illegal. I was also advised by a policeman friend that parents who serve or allow alcohol to be served to their children's friends in their homes are subject to a fine or imprisonment. If a youngster leaves under the influence of alcohol and is involved in an alcohol-related automobile accident and kills or injures someone else while driving drunk, the parent who served the alcohol can be held liable for the accident and could face a civil suit.

If a child does come home drunk, a parent should make sure that the young person is physically safe. If the child is ill (nauseated, vomiting) or incoherent (disoriented, confused), the parent should seek medical attention. When the child is sober, the parents should discover the circumstances under which the alcohol was served. The parent shoulds calmly explain that they will be observing the child's behavior more closely and that they have developed some guidelines for making sure that the child adheres to these stipulated rules. The child and the parents should discuss alternative activities so that the young person might be able to avoid use of and intoxication from alcohol in the future. Above all, parents must try not to get angry and should avoid constantly reminding the child of his/her mistake as time goes on.

To avoid death from injuries related to alcohol abuse—whether they be auto accidents, falls, or whatever—prevention is the key. We have to be observant of our own children and also work within the community to get programs in place that can help all children make rational choices about alcohol. Parents, as a last resort, have to find ways of preventing teens from driving while intoxicated.

If these measures do not prevent reoccurring abuse of alcohol and other drugs, parents should be aware that there are changes that will be evident in the child's behavior over time. If the signs of a budding addiction are known, parents can perhaps intervene before fatal consequences occur. Typically, one or both parents will note a change in the child's disposition. The teen may appear more irritable, depressed, and hostile, while responsibility for chores and school work begins to wane. Teenagers may have new friends, dress differently, stay out later more frequently, be much more difficult to communicate with, and be more secretive about their activities. There may be physical and mental changes that make them less able to function. Teen behavior may become more and more difficult for parents to tolerate, or these young people may be careless and leave evidence of their growing addiction strewn about the house. Sometimes the desperate and troubled children borrow or steal money or take other things from home that can be pawned or sold for quick cash. They may get into trouble with the law for shoplifting or drug use. Ultimately, these kids may think about or even attempt suicide.

Alert and watchful parents cannot help but notice these changes in their children. Yet so often it happens that behavioral shifts are not observed or noticed. Frequently the unusual behavior is observed but parents don't know that it signals trouble. So controlling alcohol and drug abuse begins with an alert parent or a concerned adult. The typical illegal street drugs used by teens—marijuana or "crack" cocaine—produce changes similar to alcohol. Teens using illegal, mind-altering drugs on a frequent basis almost always have discipline problems in school and experience physical and mental changes that affect their ability to conduct normal daily life. As their addiction to drugs becomes more entrenched, many teenagers end up dealing to support their habit. And we have already discussed their willingness to steal to procure the money needed to maintain a constant drug supply. Parents, take the time to look for these changes in your child, and seek help both for yourselves and your teen as soon as possible. School psychologists or counselors are good sources for information and guidance. A family physician or clergyman can often suggest alternatives available in the parents' community.

Obviously, whether it be illegal drugs or alcohol, we have to find ways to curtail their availability to our children. This has become an overwhelming task for communities throughout the country. To combat the deliberate efforts of drug pushers to recruit our kids, parents have to be alert to changes in their neighborhood and the community at large. Adults must work to prevent early involvement with drugs; education programs and public awareness campaigns are great ways to increase the level of community support for keeping children drug free. There are many organizations that can help parents develop community support systems. It's every parent's obligation to educate themselves about what *they* can do and what's available in their area.

The importance of looking so closely at the abuse of drugs and alcohol among our children is that these are the ultimate culprits in a great many teen accidents, injuries, and deaths. These substances also seem related to the increasing homicide rates for this age group. Therefore, parents must wage their own war of drug education and awareness in every family, every neighborhood, every community, and throughout the nation. The problem is too widespread not to look at all these changes with an open mind.

Confronting Domestic and Neighborhood Violence

We have already discussed accidents during the teen years, but we should also consider the violence to which teenagers are exposed. It is hard to protect our children from all the potential sources of harm out there in the real world, but we parents can give our kids some protection. First of all, each of us must really look at our own family. Even if we do everything we can for our teenagers, is the home a happy one? Does an adult or parent have a drug or drinking problem? Is there marital discord or are there frequent arguments in the home that make the environment uncomfortable for a developing child? Are the parents involved in domestic violence? Is the mother a "battered" wife? Children can be exposed to and victimized by such violence at any point in their growing years. It is important to examine the home environment, because if there are many family problems, they can force our teenagers to spend their time roaming the streets or force them out of the home entirely as runaways or victims of abandonment.

As parents, we can become so preoccupied with our own lives, jobs, problems, and relationships that we may not be aware of their individual or collective impact on our own behavior, on our home lives, or on the depth of attention we give to our children's problems. It is important to examine these dynamics of family living because children from homes where there is a great deal of stress tend to be more prone to accidents. Additionally, if there is family discord, there may also be family violence with potentially lethal consequences for the children. If family problems are apparent, they must be faced and help or counseling sought. If teenagers are exposed to a parent who is a drug or alcohol abuser, they will need support in dealing with the resulting anger and frustration that frequently is evidenced in their behavior. If this anxiety goes unattended, teenagers may vent this hostility elsewhere and engage in activities that potentially put them at risk. Again, children who come from families where there are many problems often have difficulty with their own self-esteem.

Lack of self-esteem may encourage teenagers to take dangerous risks while outside the home just to get approval and acceptance from friends or peers. Children who find themselves unable to deal with problems at home often run away, at which point they are even more at risk for potential violence and harm. These young people can be exploited or used by adults who are more "street smart." In such tragic situations, many runaways turn to prostitution or drug dealing to support themselves. If you are the parent of a runaway, be aware that organizations exist that can help you and your child (see Appendix A).

Teenagers in urban settings often gain a sense of family when they enter gang-type organizations. These gangs are frequently violent and exert tremendous influence on a teen to cooperate in illegal and dangerous activities. In some rough neighborhoods a child's very survival may mean being a member of a gang against his or her will. Parents, concerned adults, and law-enforcement officials in every community, whether large or small, must work together to confront and eliminate the violence found in gang activities. Parents, however, have to make sure their home is a safe and peaceful place for a child. Otherwise, their teens may seek out these dangerous groups or simply run away.

Based on the experiences of the young female runaway I spoke of earlier (chapter 2), life as a child who flees from home is fraught with danger. Shelters exist but they have very limited funds and facilities, and may not be able to cope with the large number of children who run away each year. Therefore, many kids find other more potentially deadly methods to survive—and many ultimately become death statistics. According to Senator Paula Hawkins in her book *Children at Risk,* 11 percent of the children who voluntarily leave home end up victims of criminal or sexual exploitation. As parents, then, we must face problems at the home front; if we don't, our children's self-esteem and well-being could be threatened and the risk of teen flight could increase dramatically. We then become powerless to shield our children from street violence. If there is violence in the home, then parents must care enough for their kids to seek the necessary counseling to help relieve the problem. Yes, counseling does cost money and many families are unable to pay for it, but even if a parent does not have the funds, there are organizations or crisis centers that can offer advice and literature on parent and teenage relationships. Some government counseling centers base their fees on the client's ability to pay. As citizens, we cannot forget the ravages of poverty on the teen years and the potential for getting involved with the wrong crowd. We also must remember that abuse and neglect during earlier years may make our children more vulnerable to violence and prone to criminal activities during the teenage years. Poverty breeds violence.

Recognizing the Signs of Potential Suicide

Suicide is yet another major killer of teenagers and young adults, especially white males. The statistics discussed in chapter 5 indicate that suicide has been a major problem in the United States and threatens to be an even bigger problem in the next decade. Again, parents must be alert to this danger, but society must be willing to ensure that family and individual support systems will be available and will have adequate resources to respond to children at risk.

The son of a neighbor of mine committed suicide in high school. He hanged himself. I asked my neighbor if she would share her insights about what changes occurred in her son Rod before the suicide; her recollections might help other parents to see the danger signs in their own children.

She first noticed that something might be wrong when Rod, a good student, started to receive poor grades. At one point, she was called by the school about her son's repeated absences over the past several months. He also seemed more distant, and appeared to dress carelessly. Having been the type of young man who was conscious of his appearance, Rod became less careful, over a period of time, about personal hygiene. He seemed depressed at times, but when approached about it he said he was just upset about going off to college and leaving his girlfriend and buddies behind. Rod eventually became forgetful about chores around the house, stayed mostly in his room, and became violent when asked to do anything out of the ordinary. Normally, a respectful and quiet kid, Rod had a fight with a next-door neighbor over his dog and was very abusive and threatening. The neighbor neglected to tell the mother until after the young man had died, because of their long-term friendship.

After Rod's death, everyone who had known him could point out behavioral changes, but no one at the time really believed that he could kill himself. The changes did not occur overnight; that fact might have made it harder to see them. However, Rod's angry outbursts over trivial matters had been going on for some time. His mother didn't believe that it was anything but a passing phase and thought these behavioral changes would disappear as he matured. Unfortunately, Rod did not get the therapy he so desperately needed. The school counselor had met with him about his grades, but Rod succeeded in convincing the counselor that he was having a temporary problem and that soon it would change for the better. Because he had always been a very good student, the counselor took Rod at his word. The counselor did recommend therapy if Rod continued to have problems, and unfortunately, the school and the parents did not communicate very well. The end result was a tragic suicide.

During this frustrating period, Rod's mother was having problems at work, so many of her son's distress signals were not as noticeable to her. Afterwards, she found out that her son had been heartbroken over a breakup with his girlfriend. There was evidence in his belongings that he had also begun using drugs on a regular basis. The changes in his behavior might seem obvious looking back, but they weren't to her at the time. This is just one case but it is not unlike many taking place throughout the country.

Other parents can learn from this personal tragedy: zero in on any changes in your child's attitudes and behavior. If a noticeable change occurs, talk with your children—listen to what they say. Relate your concern about these behavior shifts in nonjudgmental terms and, above all, get counseling for your child. The school counselor, your clergyman, or a physician can recommend help for your troubled teen.

The most common factor in adolescent suicide is the lack or loss of a meaningful relationship. Subtle references to suicide as well as obvious attempts at self-destruction should be explored by concerned parents and adults. Young boys may express depression by dangerous acts, whereas girls are more often inclined to make suicidal threats or gestures. All may express feelings of helplessness or hopelessness. Children who have experienced the loss of a meaningful relationship or seem to lack this type of relationship in their lives are particularly at risk. Parents must always work to make sure that their children feel good about themselves.

Every citizen can help save our children by ensuring that all who work with teenagers and young adults are very aware of the distress signals that indicate suicidal tendencies. Many cities have outreach programs for this high-risk group. In addition, a number of schools and colleges have anonymous suicide hot lines or counseling centers. Some communities have counseling services available with sliding scale fees based on income. However, parents are the front line; they must be tuned in to their children. They must communicate and listen to their teenager's problems. If a child threatens suicide or makes homicidal threats, immediate help is needed.

WHAT THE COMMUNITY CAN DO

As parents and as citizens, we can help prevent many teenage deaths. The following measures would go a long way toward eliminating the causes of these unnecessary deaths:

1. Begin early to teach children about alcohol and drug abuse. We should make rules about their use and abide by them ourselves.

2. Support efforts at the grade school, high school, or community level for educational programs about substance abuse. Also, be willing to invest time and energy in these programs.

3. Recognize the signs of drug and alcohol addiction and be prepared to react in a constructive way when they are observed in our children.

4. Provide treatment and counseling centers that are prepared to deal with teenage drug and alcohol abuse and addiction.

5. Ensure that our children have a peaceful home in which they can grow and develop. If there are family problems, seek all available help to cope with or correct them.

6. Recognize the signs and symptoms of potential suicide; be prepared to react quickly and effectively when these signs are exhibited by a teenager.

7. Educators and other professionals who deal with teenagers and young adults should be conscious of the danger signs of suicide and knowledgeable about how to act and react when they are noticed in children.

8. At teen parties and functions make sure that good alternatives to drinking are available.

9. Launch mass-media and educational programs to ensure that driving drunk is discouraged among our nation's youth. We need

to create new and exciting programs that work to decrease this deadly activity among our teenagers.

10. Find ways to deal with the violence associated with drugs and gang-type activities. Most references indicate that good communication and supervision at home can curtail participation in gangs. The entire community must work together to combat this serious threat to our teenagers.

11. Find ways to reduce the number of teenage runaways. The fact that young people run away places them at higher risk for exploitation and violence on the streets.

12. High-risk young-people's programs should be developed and centrally administered to provide coordinated services to the teen populations stricken by the ravages of poverty and violence.

13. Parents with few if any social support mechanisms (e.g., single mothers of lower socio-economic status) should be provided with publicly funded programs so they in turn can learn how to help their children develop or increase self-esteem.

14. Strategies should be improved to provide increased outreach and service delivery in public-health settings to promote family planning and to reduce teen pregnancy.

15. African-Americans continue to have a larger number of childhood deaths than their white counterparts. Steps must be taken to reduce this figure.

16. We must confront the harsh realities of sociocultural, economic, and political factors that have curtailed services to our less fortunate teenage populations.

17. It is important to examine the services that currently exist and find out why they are failing our youth.

Part Six

Conclusion

14

Beginning the Campaign to Save Our Children

Why are our children dying? It seems quite simple: in many situations we are letting them die. Parents, the adult population, and our social support mechanisms are not doing enough to prevent thousands of unnecessary fatalities each year. Even in those cases where childhood death is simply not preventable—i.e., when children contract diseases for which there are no known cures—we must be willing to fund the research to eradicate them. However, it has been reported that almost 80 percent of the deaths in children *could be avoided*. These senseless fatalities are what should concern us most, for this is the territory where parents and concerned adults can and must intervene if our children are to be protected. We owe them that, don't we?

Many types of accidents are preventable and yet they claim the lives of children across every age group. The type of fatal accident may differ depending upon the age of the child, but the bottom line is that many of these accidents can be avoided if adequate supervision and care is taken. We adults must be aware of the causes of these accidents and devise systems to prevent their occurrence. But do parents really know the primary causes of childhood death in their own communities? The information I have drawn upon is national in perspective, but in any community the primary causes of accidental death may vary slightly. It is important that parents become concerned members of their community and in so doing get a handle on the specific problems facing the youth where they live. With this knowledge in hand, special programs can be created and expanded to address and if possible reduce the startling rise in accidental injury and death. If there aren't any appropriate programs or services, then parents must become activists, working with local officials until there are preventive measures in place that will help decrease the number of children falling victim to accidental death.

We know, for example, that falls result in the untimely deaths of many children under the age of one year. For those aged one to four and five to nine, fires and drownings are killing thousands nationally. How does *your* community or neighborhood compare with these statistics? What is *your* community doing to curtail and prevent these types of accidental deaths? You may think you're powerless to do anything about the risks to young lives, but you're not! One person can often spearhead an entire movement. History abounds with examples of concerned citizens who have made a difference. We cannot be complacent about these deaths. There are agencies in the community that can help, but they need committed parents and adult volunteers if they are to succeed. By being knowledgeable about your community's needs and the resources available, you can at least begin to build on this solid foundation: gaps in the available resources can be noted so that new services can be created to meet the needs of the children in the community.

Educating parents and the community to the hazards facing our children in their environment is essential. For example, if there are signficant numbers of deaths related to bicycle or swimming accidents in your community, what programs currently exist to address and prevent future accidents? If none is available, talk to school and civic leaders to see if specific activities can be developed that would focus on the problems and help reduce the number of injuries or fatalities. Look at the specific causes of these deaths. Does a persistent pattern emerge? Are the circumstances of the deaths similar? Use your political clout—your vote and your membership in organizations—to get answers and to seek remedies. Public awareness may be the key: many people are not sure whether programs exist to address the problems they face as children or grownups. The community as a whole may not even be aware of a problem or the causes of certain childhood accidents. Parents and adults may not know which types of accidents are the most frequent factors in the deaths of their young people. A basic approach would incorporate the following:

1. Determine the major causes of accidental injuries and deaths involving children in your community.

2. Identify what resources and programs are currently available to prevent the recurrence of these accidents/deaths.

3. Once you identify the programs, determine if they are available in your community and what they actually provide.

4. Try to determine whether community members are aware of the accidents/conditions that cause problems and the services available to prevent them.

5. Find other parents interested in the project and work with community leaders to modify existing programs. Make the public aware of services that could potentially reduce fatalities, and/or develop new ones if need be.

6. Work to create greater public awareness of the risks plaguing our young people and the programs that could help to save our children. Keep abreast of new services as they emerge. Child safety must be our major concern. If accidents, injuries, and deaths are the result of ignorance, we must be educated about the causes. If they are a result of negligence, we must have systems in place that protect vulnerable children. Every caring adult should work toward developing solutions rather than wait for someone else to solve these problems. Parents and adults must do this for the children, since they are ill-prepared to do it for themselves.

Parents and adults need to examine the impact of pressing social problems on the community: teenage pregnancy, drug and alcohol abuse, child abuse and neglect, and suicide. What can *we* do to decrease the number of fatalities related to the above situations? Again, we must look at available community programs designed to deal with these particular problems, the effectiveness of these programs, and the community awareness of both the problems and the current options for ending the destruction of innocent lives.

One of the individuals whom I previously interviewed, told me about a school board that would not allow a teenage counseling center to be located within the high school. This center could have provided much needed information on sex education, birth control, and sexually transmitted disease. It could have provided free testing and referral services. The situation in that community is not unlike those faced in many parts of the country. Teenage pregnancy is at epidemic levels; many parents in that community were trying to find a workable solution to a problem they perceived as affecting their community. It was indeed a problem, and after much debate the parents in that community eventually succeeded in having counseling services placed in their high school. Their activism and persistence paid off.

This is one solution but not the only one. Parents and community agencies have to work within their available resources. However, sometimes these resources and services can be modified to better meet the needs of the population. In my own community I was surprised to find a number of programs and servcies of which I was unaware, even though I work in the health-care field. Parents and indeed all concerned and caring adults need to take on the responsibility of finding out what's available to meet the needs of children in their community. If a program or service does not meet the community's expectations, then citizens should voice their concerns so that steps are taken to modify the service until it is an effective resource for the children who need it. A drug or alcohol education project that touches a small segment of the population may look good on paper, but it is not an effective solution to this overwhelming problem.

Ensuring that programs and policies are sensitive to the needs of the community implies not only that the citizenry be familiar with and active in the programs but that concerned voters take an active interest in the politics surrounding these programs for children. Parents have every right to demand to know the effectiveness of a particular child welfare program and to question the government about services that exist for their children. Once the questioning and examining begins, perhaps the duplication of services will be noted and rectified. We my find that consolidating services to children will ensure that more of the money allocated to these programs is spent on actual services rather than being consumed by administrative costs and overlapping programs. Parents should get the maximum benefit from the tax dollars they spend. If need be, a public outcry for services that benefit our children may be in order. This is well within our rights as citizens and as parents.

Perhaps the most important role we have as parents and adults is as child advocates, who actively work to promote the interests not only of our own children but of *all* children. Parents and concerned citizens alike must concentrate on the deplorable conditions that exist for a growing segment of our population. We know that the money available for welfare and Medicaid is inadequate to protect fully the children of poverty. Let us work more diligently to promote better funding for these programs and to raise the minimum wage requirements. We must be certain that the funding provided to the poor never again falls far below minimal living standards. The health-care provision to poor children must be adequate and good prenatal care has to be available to poor pregnant women.

Furthermore, programs such as WIC should always have full support. According to the Children's Defense Fund (1989), only 40 percent of those eligible for this program are being served. Finally, we should ensure that immunization programs, Head Start preschool programs, and the Job Corps for disadvantaged youth are expanded.

The Children's Defense Fund (1989) has stated how much the nation could save by investing in these programs rather than saving now only by postponing the consequences of neglecting poor children until the situation grows worse decades down the road. This organization believes that there are various ways we as parents can help poor children. Its survey suggests that America's adult population wants more programs for children and is willing to allocate more government funds to these programs to ensure that all children get an equal opportunity. Many of these polls have shown that citizens are also willing to pay more taxes to subsidize such programs if necessary. Here are some additional steps that the Fund suggests be taken: First, we should write to our federal and state officials and representatives pressuring them to put child welfare issues near the top of their priority list. Second, local officials should be invited to community forums where children's issues can be discussed and addressed. Third, we should visit children's programs and become more familiar with those that exist in our communities. Additionally, within civic and social clubs, we can use monies collected from fundraising to help subsidize children's programs that aid needy children rather than just supporting social functions for our group. On a personal level, each of us should get involved with the children in our area and offer guidance wherever and however we can. If we all joined groups that provide services to needy children, many of the problems that affect young lives could be addressed. The Children's Defense Fund provides a great deal of information on programs implemented at the local level that have been successful in meeting the needs of poor children. The success of these programs usually involves a committed community that really addresses the problems of their neediest citizens.

Parents and involved citizens throughout America must work hard to reduce child fatalities. It's our problem. We must find the solution, and the key ingredients are our involvement, commitment, awareness, and activism with regard to child welfare issues. It is time that the American adult population move as a unified front to combat the dangers surrounding our children. By investing in our kids and preserving their health and safety, we preserve ourselves, our history, our future, and our nation. The children *must* be our national priority in the years ahead. Our first step is awareness, our second step is knowledge, but the crucial step is action. Can we afford to delay any longer?

Afterword

What follows is one woman's description of her struggle to safeguard her family after the death of her husband.

How does it feel to lose a child? So many people have asked me that question. I grew to hate it, always thinking there must be something wrong with me. I became a widow at thirty-four, left to become mother, father, provider, educator, and all else that it takes two parents to do. Be a disciplinarian, balance the checkbook, wash the clothes, cook, get the kids to school, help with homework and more and more and more. Then the big question, how? Oh, you hear how there is so much help. Twenty odd years later, I ask again, where? I never found the answers.

To go back a little, I was brought up in a good, solid, middle-class family. I knew right from wrong. I was always honest and trusting. I believed in the adage "Show me your company and I'll tell you what you are." I went to church on Sunday and said my prayers at night. I believed in marriage and big families. When I grew to be an adult, I had a wonderful marriage and seven beautiful children. For a number of years, this pattern continued. I was a solid, honest, and upstanding citizen—and then it all changed. A sequence of events occurred that changed my life forever and made me realize that life in this country could be as cruel as it had been good.

When my husband died, I remembered sitting on my porch thinking, "What do I do now?" A "thoughtful" in-law at the funeral told me that I would probably lose my children since I had no means of support now that my husband was dead. He told me they would probably be better off in foster care. When I sought help for myself and my children, there was little help for me. My husband's illness left me deeply in debt. If I wanted welfare, I would have to sign over my house. It was the only thing I had left after my husband's illness. I could obtain limited health insurance but it would never be enough for all my children and myself. I was eligible for social security and a veterans pension. Surely, that was going to help. If I accepted that help, I couldn't earn over a certain amount, and the amount given to me was not enough to support my children. So I began working under the table to make ends meet. For the first time in my life I became a crook. My children had to help and had to care for themselves.

My beautiful six-year-old daughter was struck by a drunk driver on her way home from school, a block away from her safe, fenced yard. My two older children, who were walking with her, witnessed this horror. My son, who tried to grab her, was also hit and thrown into a nearby tree. He survived, but my daughter did not. I wished I could have climbed into their minds and erased that horror; maybe I could have helped. But in my own grief, I forgot all else. No one offered me help. No one told me I needed help. I got pity, a beautiful funeral mass, and a lovely headstone. The driver went free. No one ever tested him for alcohol intoxication. He was a pillar of the community—no one questioned his actions. It was my child who was at fault—she didn't get across the street fast enough. Never mind that the driver was speeding on the wrong side of the road.

I had no one to care for my children, and I could not afford help. In desperation, I seriously thought of killing myself. There seemed no way out of this. I kept working; I tried to get an education. I often had to pull my sixteen-year-old daughter out of school to care for the other kids. I could not bear another tragedy!

I remember there were times when my children and I ate cereal and nothing else for days because it was the only thing left in the house. I kept working and being paid under the table so that I could exist. I was poor and getting poorer every day. My whole life became a game of survival. My children paid the ultimate price; they had lost their father and, in a way, their mother. Would my six-year-old have died if I had the type of job where I could leave and pick her up? I had no choice and the system gave me no choice. My six-year-old is not the only fatality. My other children survived but the home environment left a lot to be desired. My heart broke because my sixteen-year-old never finished school. My children all left school eventually, disheartened and beaten.

You can't tell me this great nation helped me. I was alone and did the best I could. I survived and raised my children. With a little support, my children would all have done better. With a little help, perhaps my six-year-old would have survived. I do feel she was a victim of a system that didn't care. It seems a cruel irony to me that a system that cannot support and protect a little child like my daughter could support and protect the drunk who killed her. I wasn't a mother who didn't care. I was simply a mother who couldn't care. My children were all victims.

Anonymous

This is a fitting note with which to end our discussion because it summarizes a number of points I have been making throughout. This woman's struggle to raise her family was compounded by the lack of social support given to her. Her options were few. In her heart, the guilt over her child's death haunts her. The lack of child-care options is a real factor for any poor mother. They do not have the wide range of choices that most of us enjoy. The bitter struggle for survival should not have to be endured in a prosperous nation. This story also points out the thin line separating the "good life" from poverty. What happened to this prosperous, middle-class woman could happen to any of us. It is not a distant possibility but a distinct, very real one. It also points out the vulnerability of our children to situations well beyond their control. The mother's point about the system that would not provide enough support for her to care for her child is poignant and illustrative of our indifference to children and to their safety. It's time that we speak clearly and decisively as a nation: Our children are dying before our eyes—and only an organized effort will stop the carnage! We can do it. But are we willing to make the sacrifices to save our kids? Each of us will have to look inside himself for the answer.

Appendix A

What follows is a listing of organizations and/or referral services that parents can contact for additional help and information. Check your local telephone directory for agencies or offices corresponding to those listed here for New York State.

Alcoholics Anonymous—
   World Services
P.O. Box 459
Grand Central Station
New York, NY 10163
(212) 686-1100
*(AA is listed in most telephone
   directories)*

Al-Anon Family Group
   Headquarters, Inc.
P.O. Box 862 Midtown Station
New York, NY 10018
(212) 302-7240

Allstate
Dept. 500
P.O. Box 7600
Mt. Prospect, IL 60056-9961
*Will provide a free pamphlet by the
   American Academy of Pediat-
   rics and a discount coupon
   from Sears on child car seats.*

American Humane Association
9725 East Hampden Avenue
Denver, CO 80231
(303) 695-0811
*Offers training/information on
   child welfare and child
   protection.*

Big Brothers/Big Sisters
230 N. 13th Street
Philadelphia, PA 19107
(215) 567-7000
*Matches children with adult
    volunteers who serve as special
    friends or role models.*

Child Abuse Prevention
    Information Resources Center
134 South Swan Street
Albany, NY 12210
(800) 342-7472*
*State-wide information and referral
    regarding child abuse preven-
    tion and family issues.*

Child Abuse and Maltreatment
    Reporting Center
40 North Pearl Street
Albany, NY 12243
(800) 342-3720
*Child abuse and maltreatment
    register. Available services 7
    days a week, 24 hours a day.*

Child Find, Inc.
P.O. Box 277
New Platz, NY 12561
(800) 426-5678
*Registers missing children and
    offers counseling to runaways.*

Child Help's National Child Abuse
    Hotline
Child Help USA
P.O. Box 630
Hollywood, CA 90028

(800) 422-4453
*Crisis information referral service
    dealing with child abuse in all
    fifty states.*

Child Welfare League of America
440 First Street, N.W.
Washington, DC 20001
(202) 638-2952
*Consulting and training for public
    and private welfare agencies.*

Children of Alcoholics
    Foundation, Inc.
P.O. Box 4185
Grand Central Station
New York, NY 10163
(212) 351-2680

Children's Rights of America, Inc.
12551 Indian Rocks Road, Suite 9
Largo, FL 34644
(800) 442-4673
(800) 874-1111
*Counseling hotline for parents with
    a missing child.*

Domestic Violence Hotline
Women's Building
79 Central Avenue
Albany, NY 12206
(800) 942-6906
*State-wide referral service dealing
    with domestic violence.*

---

*All 800 numbers are toll-free

Drug Abuse Information Line
Pride-Site Information Hot Line
371 East 10th Street
New York, NY 10009
(800) 522-5353
*State-wide information and referral
agency dealing with drug abuse
and offering other services.*

Hospicelink
Essex Square, Suite 3B
Essex, CT 06426
(800) 331-1620
*Supplies general information and
referrals to programs nationwide for the terminally ill.*

MADD
Mothers Against Drunk Driving
National Processing Center
P.O. Box 541688
Dallas, TX 75354-1688
(214) 744-6233

Missing Children (Kidwatch)
    Hotline (24 hrs.)
(800) 451-9422

National Association for Children
    of Alcoholics
31582 Coast Highway, Suite B
South Laguna, CA 92677
(714) 499-3889

National Association of Counsel
    for Children
1205 Oneida Street
Denver, CO 80220
(303) 321-3963
Serves attorneys who represent

*children. Offers information on
legislative developments on
children's issues.*

National Center for Missing and
    Exploited Children
2101 Wilson Blvd., Suite 550
Arlington, VA 22201
(800) 843-5678
(202) 634-9821
*Toll free number is for parents of
missing children. Regular number is for information and
referral.*

National Child Safety Counsel
4065 Page Avenue
Michigan Center, MI 49254
(517) 764-6070
*Provides law enforcement agencies
and schools with safety
education materials for children.*

National Clearinghouse for Alcohol
    and Drug Information
P.O. Box 2345
Rockville, MD 20852
(301) 468-2600
*Provides information on alcohol
and drug-related topics.*

National Clearinghouse on Child
    Abuse and Neglect Information
U.S. Department of Health and
    Human Services
P.O. Box 1182
Washington, DC 20013
(703) 821-2086
*National resource for information
on all aspects of child abuse.*

National Coalition for Children's
  Justice
2119 Shelburne Road
Shelburne, VT 05482
(802) 985-8458
*Dedicated to improving protective
  services to the young and
  creating public awareness of
  social injustices to children.*

National Committee for the
  Prevention of Child Abuse
322 South Michigan Avenue
Suite 1600
Chicago, IL 60604
(312) 663-3520
*Works for the prevention of child
  abuse and neglect through
  public awareness programs.
  State chapters and
  informational materials.*

National Conference of State
  Legislatures
1056 17th Street, Suite 2100
Denver, CO 80265
(303) 623-7800
*Provides information to state
  legislatures and their staffs.*

National Council of Juvenile and
  Family Court Judges
P.O. Box 8970
Reno, NV 89507
(702) 784-6012
*Provides training for judges in
  juvenile and family courts.*

National Crime Prevention Council
1700 K Street N.W., Suite 2006
Washington, DC 20006
(202) 466-6272
*Produces national advertising
  campaigns to reduce crime.*

National Institute on Alcohol
  Abuse and Alcoholism
5600 Fishers Lane
Rockville, MD 20857
(301) 443-3885

National Institute for Latchkey
  Children
P.O. Box 682
Glen Echo, MD 20812
(301) 229-6126
*Provides resources available in par-
  ent's local area for latchkey
  kids.*

NYS Consumer Protection Board
Complaint Unit
State Consumer Protection Board
99 Washington Avenue
Albany, NY 12210
(518) 474-8583
*Consumer advisors are available to
  answer questions from 8:30 to
  11:00 A.M. and from 3:00 to
  5:00 P.M. All complaints must
  be submitted in writing.*

ODPHP National Health
  Information Center
P.O. Box 1133
Washington, D.C. 20013-1133
(800) 336-4797
Refers callers to national

*organizations that deal with a
variety of health topics. (Does
not diagnose symptoms.)*

Parents Anonymous
6733 South Spulveda Blvd.
Suite 270
Los Angeles, CA 90045
(800) 421-0353
*Offers free group or one-to-one
support for abusive parents as
well as a telephone hotline to
help parents cope with child
rearing.*

Parents Without Partners
8807 Colesville Road
Silverspring, MD 20910
(301) 588-9354 (9355)
*Offers support, social events, and
family activities for single
parents.*

PRIDE (Parent Resource Institute
Drug Education)
Hurt Building, Suite 210
50 Hurt Plaza
Atlanta, GA 30303
(800) 241-7946
*Teaches prevention of drug abuse
through education.*

Save Our Selves (SOS)
Secular Organizations for Sobriety
Box 5
Buffalo, NY 14215
(716) 834-2921
*Provides an alternative, secular
recovery method for alcoholics
and drug addicts who are
uncomfortable with the
spiritual content of widely
available twelve-step programs.*

TOUGHLOVE
P.O. Box 1069
Doylestown, PA 18901
(215) 348-7090
*Groups across the United States
offer special help to parents
who have troubled and/or
difficult teenagers.*

U.S. Consumer Product Safety
Commission
Washington, D.C. 20207
(800) 638-2772
*National agency that provides
safety-related information
about products used in and
around the home. This agency
will also receive consumer complaints on home products such
as toys, etc.*

Appendix B

BOOKLETS AVAILABLE FREE:

BROCHURE NAME
DEPARTMENT C
American Academy of Pediatrics
P.O. Box 927
Elk Grone Village, IL 60009-0927

(Send a separate, self-addressed business size envelope for each brochure.)

a. "You and Your Pediatrician: Common Childhood Problems"
b. "Your Child's Growth: Developmental Milestones"
c. "Surviving: Coping with Adolescent Depression and Suicide"
d. "Alcohol: Your Child and Drugs"
e. "Marijuana: Your Child and Drugs"
f. "Cocaine: Your Child on Drugs"

ADDITIONAL REFERENCES:

The U.S. Government Printing Office publishes a catalog entitled: *New Books—Publications for Sale by the Government Printing Office*. The titles listed pertain to children and appear in the June 1990 issue. They can be purchased by contacting: The Superintendent of Documents, U.S. Government Printing Office, Washington, D.C. 20402.

Report of the Secretary's Task Force on Youth Suicide
   Volume 1: *Overview and Recommendations.* 1989.
   S/N 017-024-01372-2

   Volume 2: *Risk Factors for Youth Suicide.* 1989.
   S/N 017-024-01373-1

   Volume 3: *Prevention and Interventions in Youth Suicide.* 1989.
   S/N 017-024-01374-9

   Volume 4: *Strategies for the Prevention of Youth Suicide.* 1989.
   S/N 017-024-01375-7

Experiences in School Improvement: Story of 16 American Districts. 1988.
   S/N 065-000-00343-1 (ED.1.2: Sch 6/10)

When Cocaine Affects Someone You Love. 1989.
   (Sold in packages of 100 copies.)
   S/N 017-024-01371-4

Infant Care. 1989.
   S/N 017-091-00241-0

National Adoption Directory. 1989.
   S/N 017-092-00103-7

How to Help Your Children Achieve in School. 1983.
   S/N 065-000-00176-4

Your Child From One to Six. 1978.
   S/N 017-091-00219-3

Employers and Child Care: Benefiting Work and Family. 1989.
   S/N 029-002-00076-2

   The United States General Services Administration publishes a variety of free or low-cost booklets on health and other consumer issues. A catalog entitled *Consumer Information Catalog* published by the staff of the Consumer Information Center of the General Services Administration is in many libraries (U.S. Government Printing Office, 1990, 262-868/00003). A partial list of those booklets that pertain to children appears below. *Please consult the above catalog for instructions on how to order these booklets.*

AIDS and the Education of Our Children: A Guide for Parents and Teachers
Chew or Snuff is Real Bad Stuff
Choosing a School for Your Child
Clearing the Air: A Guide to Quitting Smoking
A Consumer's Guide to Mental Health Services
Consumer's Resource Handbook
Co-op Education
Diet, Nutrition and Cancer Prevention: The Good News
Dietary Guidelines Bulletins
Dietary Guidelines for Americans
Eating for Life
Food News for Consumers
Good Sources of Nutrients
Growing Up Drug Free
Handbook on Child Support Enforcement
How to Create a Kidsummit Against Drugs
Lead and Your Drinking Water
Parents Guide to Childhood Immunization
Plain Talk About Depression
Plain Talk About Mutual Help Groups
Plain Talk About Stress
Plain Talk About Wife Abuse
Schools Without Drugs
Some Facts and Myths About Vitamins
Take Action Against Drug Abuse
Useful Information on Phobias and Panic
When Someone Close Has AIDS
What to Do When a Friend is Depressed: A Guide for Students

Two general reference books which provide addresses and phone numbers for all federal and state offices, departments, and agencies are *The Federal Executive Directory* and *The State Executive Registry*. They are available from Carroll Publishing Company, Washington, D.C. (202) 333-8260.

Bibliography

AIDS Community Services of Western New York, Inc. (March 1990). "HIV Infection among Adolescents: Falling Between the Cracks of Services and Prevention." *The AIDS Newsletter,* 4(6), p. 5.

American Heart Association (1987). *Heartsaver Manual.* Dallas, Tex.: National Center, pp. 54–67.

Anderson, L. J., et al. (April 1990). "Association Between Respiratory Syncytial Virus Outbreaks and Lower Respiratory Tract Deaths of Infants and Young Children." *Journal of Infectious Diseases,* 161, pp. 640–46.

Balter, L. (January 1988). "Understanding Kids." *Ladies Home Journal,* 105(1), pp. 62–67.

Bandura, A. (1971). *Social Learning Theory.* Morristown, N.J.: General Learning Corp.

Belleck, J., and P. Bamford. (1984). *Nursing Assessment: A Multidimensional Approach.* Monterey, Calif.: Wadsworth, Inc.

Child Welfare League of America. (1986). *Testimony and Speeches 1985.* Washington, D.C.: Child Welfare League of America.

Children's Defense Fund. (1989). *A Vision for America's Children.* Washington, D.C.: Children's Defense Fund.

"The Children's Hour." (November 7, 1988). *U.S. News and World Report,* 105(8), pp. 34–70.

Church, G. J. (May 16, 1988). "Nation—The Emerging Child Care Issue." *Time,* 131(20), p. 42.

Comecci, G. D. (September 1988). "Kids, Drugs, and Alcohol." *Good Housekeeping,* 86, p. 117.

"Cornerstone Manor Nears Completion." (March/April 1990). *City Missionary,* 2(1).

"Currents—A Scary Mix of Kids and Steroids." (December 26, 1988/ January 2, 1989). *U.S. News and World Report,* 105(25), pp. 13–14.

"Current Trends: Results from the National Adolescent Student Health Survey." (March 10, 1989). *Morbidity and Mortality Weekly Report,* 38, pp. 147–50, 165–70.

Dolan, M. A., et al. (October 1989). "Three-Wheel and Four-Wheel All-Terrain Vehicle Injuries in Children." *Pediatrics,* 84, pp. 694–98.

Dolmetsch, P., and G. Mauricette. (1987). *Teens Talk about Alcohol and Alcoholism.* Garden City, N.Y.: Doubleday & Co., Inc.

Donovan, M. E. (February 1988). "Alcohol Abuse: What Your Child Should Know." *Parents,* 63(2), pp. 189–98.

Druschel, C. M., and C. B. Hale. (December 1987). "Postneonatal Mortality among Normal Birth Weight Infants in Alabama, 1980 to 1983." *Pediatrics,* 80(6), pp. 869–72.

Erickson, E. H. (1963). *Childhood and Society.* 2nd ed. New York: W. W. Norton.

"Fatal Injuries to Children—United States, 1986." (July 6, 1990). *Morbidity and Mortality Weekly Report,* 39(26), pp. 442–451.

Fingerhut, L. A., J. C. Kleinman, M. H. Malloy, and J. J. Feldman. (July/August 1988). "Injury Fatalities among Young Children." *Public Health Report,* 103(4), pp. 399–405.

Frieberg, K. L. (1987). *Human Development: A Life Span Approach.* 3rd ed. Boston: Jones and Bartlett Publishers.

"Getting Involved: What to Do When You Suspect Child Abuse." (April 1988). *Glamour,* 85(4), p. 75.

Gork, P., and D. York (1982). *TOUGHLOVE.* Garden City, N.Y.: Doubleday & Co., Inc.

Groller, I. (September 1988). "Should I Get Involved?" *Parents,* 63(9), p. 41.

Guntheroth, W. G., et al. (April 1990). "Risk of Sudden Infant Death Syndrome in Subsequent Siblings." *Journal of Pediatrics,* 116, pp. 520–24.

Hamilton, J. O., and S. B. Garland. (January 25, 1988). "Social Issues—Vaccine Programs Need a Booster Shot." *Business Week* (3035), p. 67.

Hawkins, P. (1986). *Children at Risk: My Fight against Child Abuse—A Personal Story and a Public Plea.* Bethesda, Md.: Adler & Adler.

Hechinger, G. (1984). *How to Raise a Street Smart Child: The Complete Parent's Guide to Safety on the Street and at Home.* New York: Facts on File Publications.

Herz, E. J., L. M. Olson, and J. S. Reis. (July/August 1988). "Family Planning for Teens: Strategies for Improving Outreach and Service Delivery in Public Health Settings." *Public Health Reports,* 103(4), pp. 422–30.

"Infant Mortality by Marital Status of Mother—United States, 1983." (August 3, 1990). *Morbidity and Mortality Weekly Report,* 39, pp. 521–523.

Institute of Medicine. (1985). *Preventing Low Birth Weight.* Washington, D.C.: National Academy Press.

Johnson, S. W., and L. J. Maile. (1987). *Suicide and the Schools: A Handbook for Prevention, Intervention, and Rehabilitation.* Springfield, Ill. Charles C. Thomas, Publisher.

Josselyn, I. (1971). *Adolescence.* New York: Harper & Row Publishers.

Kimmich, M. H. (1985). *America's Children—Who Cares?* Washington, D.C.: The Urban Institute Press.

Klaus, M., and J. Kennell. (1976). *Maternal-Infant Bonding.* St. Louis, Mo.: C. V. Mosby Co.

Kogan, N. (1976). *Cognitive Styles in Infancy and Early Childhood.* New York: Wiley.

Lear, J. G., H. W. Foster, Jr., and J. A. Baratz. (May 1989). "The High-Risk Young People's Program. A Summing Up." *Journal Adolescent Health Care,* 10(3), pp. 224–30.

"Low Birthweight—United States, 1975–1987." (March 8, 1990). *Morbidity and Mortality Weekly Report,* 39, pp. 148–51.

Manton, K. G., C. H. Patrick, and K. W. Johnson. (1987). "Health Differentials between Blacks and Whites: Recent Trends in Morality and Morbidity." *Milbank Quarterly* (Suppl. 1), pp. 129–99.

McCoy, K. (1987). *Solo Parenting: Your Essential Guide. How to Find the Balance between Parenthood and Personhood.* New York: New American Library.

McIntire, M. S., and C. R. Angle. (1980). *Suicide Attempts in Children and Youth.* Hagerstown, Md.: Harper & Row Publishers, Inc.

Meier, J. H. (1985). *Assault against Children.* San Diego, Calif.: College-Hill Press.

Miller, C. A., A. Fine, S. Adams-Taylor, and L. B. Schorr. (1986). *Monitoring Children's Health: Key Indicators.* Washington, D.C.: American Public Health Association.

Milo, N. (1971). *9226 Kercheval: The Storefront That Didn't Burn.* University of Michigan Press: Ann Arbor Paperbacks.

Moses, D., and R. Burger. (1975). *Are You Driving Your Children to Drink?* New York: Van Nostrand Reinhold Company.

"Mumps Prevention." (June 9, 1989). *Morbidity and Mortality Weekly Report,* 38, pp. 388–92, 397–400.

National Center for Health Statistics. (1986). *Health United States 1986 and Prevention Profile* (Department of Health and Human Services Publication No. [PHS] 87-1232). Washington, D.C.: U.S. Government Printing Office.

———. (1988). *Health United States 1988 and Prevention Profile* (Department of Health and Human Services Publication No. [PHS] 87-1232). Washington, D.C.: U.S. Government Printing Office.

———. (March 1989). *Health United States 1988.* (Department of Health and Human Services Pub. No. [PHS] 88-1232). Public Health Service, Washington, D.C.: U.S. Government Printing Office.

———. (1990). *Vital Statistics of the United States, 1987,* vol. 2, Mortality, Part A. Washington, D.C.: Public Health Service, 1990.

National Institutes of Health. (March 1988). *A Mortality Study of One Million Persons by Demographic, Social, and Economic Factors: 1979–1981 Follow-Up* (NIH Publication No. 88-2896). Washington, D.C.: U.S. Department of Health and Human Services.

New York State Council on Children and Families. (1988). *State of the Child in New York State.* Albany, N.Y.: New York State Council on Children and Families.

O'Carroll, P. W., J. A. Mercy, and J. A. Steward. (August 19, 1988). "Center for Disease Control Recommendations for a Community Plan for the Prevention and Containment of Suicide Clusters." *Morbidity and Mortality Weekly Report,* 37 (Suppl. 6), pp. 1–12.

Papalia, D. E., and S. W. Olds. (1982). *Human Development.* New York: McGraw-Hill.

Pentz, M. A., J. H. Dwyer, D. P. MacKinnon, B. R. Flay, W. B. Hansen, E. Y. Wang, and C. A. Johnson. (June 9, 1989). "A Multicommunity Trial for Primary Prevention of Adolescent Drug Abuse. Effects on Drug Use Prevalence." *Journal American Medical Association,* 261(22), pp. 3259–66.

Pfeffer, C. R. (1986). *The Suicidal Child.* New York: The Guilford Press.

Piaget, J., and B. Inhelder. (1969). *The Psychology of the Child.* New York: Basic Books.

Piggott, M. (January 6–12, 1988). "Making the Numbers Add Up." *Nursing Times,* 84(1), pp. 36–7.

Pillitteri, A. (1987). *Child Health Nursing—Care of the Growing Family.* Boston: Little, Brown and Co.

Poplack, D. G. (1985). "Acute Lymphoblastic Leukemia in Childhood." *Pediatric Clinics of North America,* 32(3), pp. 669–97.

Powell, M. (1981). *Assessment and Management of Behavioral Problems in Children.* 2nd ed. St. Louis, Mo.: C. V. Mosby Co.

"Recommendations of the Immunization Practice Advisory Committee (ACIP)—General Recommendations on Immunization." (April 7, 1989). *Morbidity and Mortality Weekly Report, 38*(13), 205–227.

Reuben, R., et al. (1977). "Adolescents Who Attempt Suicide." *Journal of Pediatrics,* p. 636.

"Rubella and Congenital Rubella Syndrome—United States, 1985–1988." (March 24, 1989). *Morbidity and Mortality Weekly Report, 38*(11), 173–178.

Ruschel, S. (1986). *Straight Talk on Drugs.* New York: King Features Syndicate, Inc.

Salk, L. (May 1988). "Dealing with Your Teenager." *Reader's Digest,* pp. 223–29.

Salvatore, D. (January 1988). "The Truth about Teens and Drinking." *Ladies Home Journal,* 105(1), pp. 68–74.

Schaefer, C. E., and H. L. Millman. (1981). *How to Help Children with Common Problems.* New York: Van Nostrand Rheinhold Company.

Schaeffer, H. R., and P. E. Emerson. (1964). "The Development of Social Attachments in Infancy." *Monographs of the Society for Research in Child Development,* p. 29.

Schulmon, S. (March 4, 1990). "Alcohol Outdoes Illegal Drugs as the Nation's Leading Killer." *Buffalo News* (Section pp. B-3 and B-4).

Servonsky, J., and S. Opas. (1987). *Nursing Management of Children.* Boston, Mass: Jones and Bartlett Publishers.

Seixas, J. S. (1979). *Alcohol: What It Is, What It Does.* New York: Greenwillow Books.

Seixas, J. S. (1987). *An Elephant in the Living Room.* Minneapolis, Minn.: CompCare Publications.

"Sex on Campus." (February 1990). *CV,* 2(1), p. 40.

Shenk, D. (February 1990). "Young Hate." *CV,* 2(1), pp. 34–39.

Smith, M. (1986). *Yes, I Can Say No—A Parent's Guide to Assertiveness Training for Children.* New York: Arbor House.

Testa, M., and F. Wulczyn. (1980). *The State of the Child—Volume One of a Series of Research Reports on Children in Illinois.* Chicago, Ill.: The Children's Policy Research Project, School of Social Service Administration, The University of Chicago.

"Unintentional Poisoning Mortality—United States, 1980–1986." (March 17, 1989). *Morbidity and Mortality Weekly Report,* 38(10), 153–157.

University Counseling Services, Division of Student Affairs, State University of New York at Buffalo (1989). *Tips on Recognizing and Dealing with Students in Emotional Distress.*

"Update: Heterosexual Transmission of Acquired Immunodeficiency Syndrome and Human Immunodeficiency Virus Infection—United States." (June 23, 1989). *Morbidity and Mortality Weekly Report,* 38, pp. 423–34.

U.S. Department of Health and Human Services/Public Health Service. (1981). *Better Health for Our Children: A National Strategy* (Vol. III and IV). Washington, D.C.: Government Printing Office.

van de Bor, M., et al. (January 1990). "Decreased Cardiac Output in Infants of Mothers Who Abused Cocaine." *Pediatrics,* 85, pp. 30–2.

VanderZanden, J. W. (1978). *Human Development.* New York: Alfred A. Knopf, Inc.

VanDyk, J. (May, 1990). "Growing Up in East Harlem." *National Geographic,* 177(5), pp. 53–75.

Wagemaker, H. (1973). *Why Can't I Understand My Kids?—Bridging the Generation Gap.* Grand Rapids, Mich.: Zondervon Corporation.

"Warning: Keep Cigarette Lighters Away from Your Child." *Glamour,* 85(4), p. 77.

Weinhaus, E., and K. Friedmon. (1988). *Stop Struggling with Your Teen.* New York: Penguin Books.

Weinhous, B. (August 1988). "How to Raise a Happy, Healthy Child." *Ladies Home Journal,* 105(8), pp. 53–70.

Weitzman, M., et al. (April 1990). "Maternal Smoking and Childhood Asthma." *Pediatrics,* 85, pp. 505–11.

Western New York Chapter Sudden Infant Death Syndrome Foundation. (1987). *Sudden Infant Death Syndrome—A Family Tragedy.*

Whaley, L., and D. Wong. (1987). *Nursing Care of Infants and Children.* St. Louis: C. V. Mosby.

Whitman, D. (November 7, 1988). "The Hollow Promise—Government Faces Big Barriers When It Comes to Helping Children." *U.S. News and World Report,* 105(8). pp. 41–44.

Whyte, L. (June 22–28, 1988). "Voluntary Organizations. Your Health Service Needs You." *Nursing Times,* 84(25), pp. 43–44.

Wieller, S. (June 1988). "Battered Children—How Can We Save Them?" *McCalls,* 115(9), pp. 57–58.

Williamson, H. A., Jr., et al. (November 1989). "Association Between Life Stress and Serious Prenatal Complication." *Journal of Family Practice,* 29, pp. 489–94.

Winn, M. (1987). *Unplugging the Plug-in Drug—Help Your Children Kick the TV Habit.* New York: Penguin Books.

Wright, L. (1980). *Parent Power—A Guide to Responsible Child-rearing.* New York: William Morrow and Company, Inc.

"Year 2000 National Health Objectives." (September 21, 1989). *Morbidity and Mortality Weekly Report,* 38, 629–33.